D0579770

total
yoga

total
yoga

nita patel

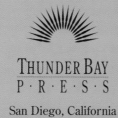

THUNDER BAY
P·R·E·S·S

San Diego, California

This book is dedicated to all who embrace truth, peace, and wisdom.
Heartfelt gratitude to my spiritual teacher, Dr. Jagjit Ram.

Thunder Bay Press

An imprint of the Advantage Publishers Group

5880 Oberlin Drive, San Diego, CA 92121-4794

www.thunderbaybooks.com

Copyright © MQ Publications 2003

Text copyright © Nita Patel 2003

Photography © page 32 Image Bank; page 166 left Science Photo Library, right Corbis; page 172
right Robert Harding Picture Library

SERIES EDITOR: Kate John, MQ Publications

EDITORIAL DIRECTOR: Ljiljana Baird, MQ Publications

PHOTOGRAPHY BY Mike Prior

DESIGN BY Balley Design Associates

ILLUSTRATION BY gerardgraphics.co.uk

Copyright under International, Pan American, and Universal Copyright Conventions. All rights
reserved. No part of this book may be reproduced or transmitted in any form or by any means,
electronic or mechanical, including photocopying, recording, or by any information storage-and-
retrieval system, without written permission from the copyright holder. Brief passages (not to exceed
1,000 words) may be quoted for reviews.

All notations of errors or omissions should be addressed to Thunder Bay Press, Editorial Department,
at the above address. All other correspondence (author inquiries, permissions) concerning the content
of this book should be addressed to MQ Publications, 12 The Ivories, 6-8 Northampton Street,
London N1 2HY, England.

ISBN 1-57145-933-2

Library of Congress Cataloging-in-Publictation Data available upon request.

Printed in China

2 3 4 5 07 06 05 04 03

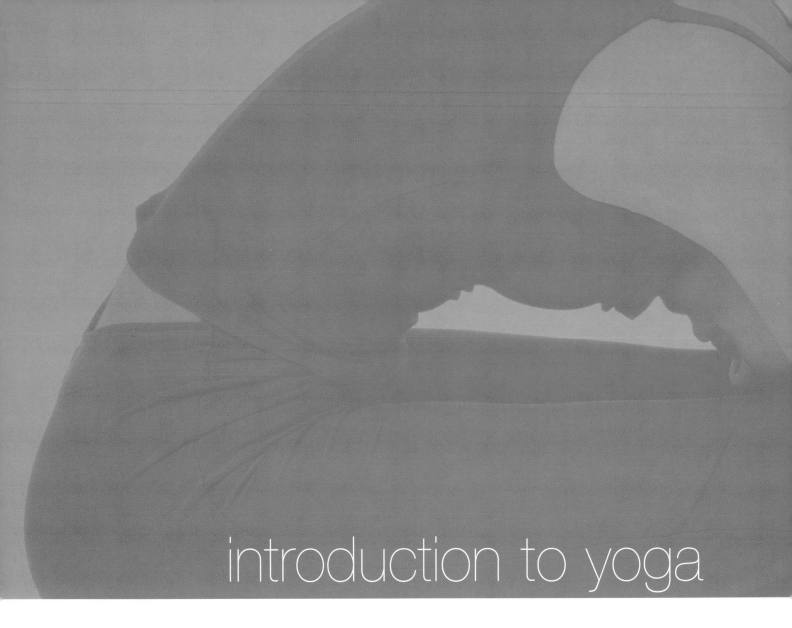

introduction to yoga

Yoga means "to yoke," "to unite," or "to be whole." Yoga is an ancient philosophical discipline, harmonizing the mind, body, and spirit. On a physical level, it enhances well-being and brings balance, strength, and vitality. For the mind, it improves memory and concentration, sharpens the intellect, and steadies the emotions to achieve a richer and more fulfilled life. On a deeper level, the practice of yoga leads to self-awareness and *moksha*, or "liberation."

Anyone can practice yoga, no matter the age, level of fitness and health, body weight, or religion. People take yoga for different reasons, but whether it is for reducing stress or toning up for a slimmer body, yoga practice will undoubtedly alter your perception of the world; it promotes physical vitality, mental serenity, and the opportunity for self-development.

This book aims to familiarize you with Hatha yoga, the science of yoga *asanas,* or postures. Over seventy asanas are featured in the form of programs for daily use. When carrying out the programs, refer back to the detailed descriptions of the asanas to ensure precise positioning. These programs can be adapted and refined to suit your own needs. Pay heed to the cautionary notes that accompany each asana. If in doubt, consult a medical practitioner to assess the suitability of the asanas. Given the intricate nature of yoga, it is advisable to practice initially under the guidance of a teacher. For more advanced yoga, a book is best used as a supplementary guide to practice.

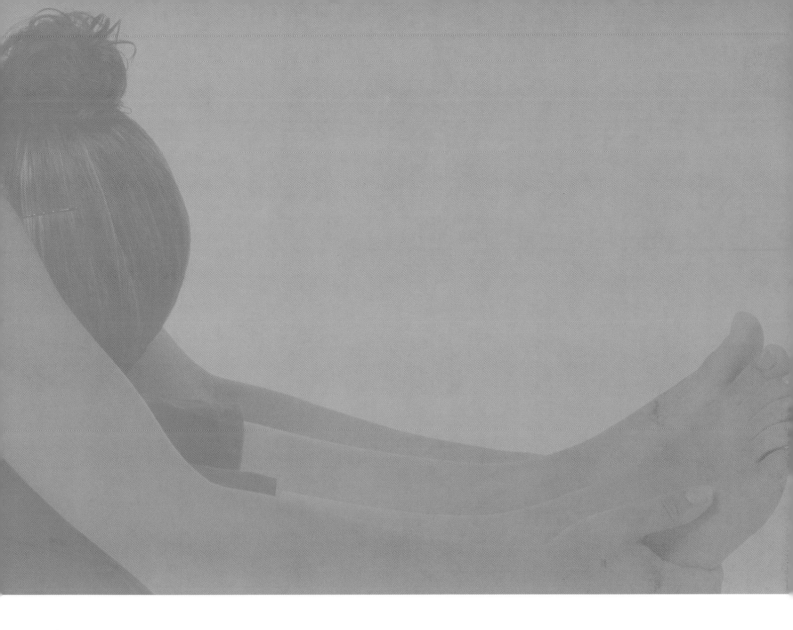

contemporary yoga

Our sophisticated technological world has relieved us of many physically demanding and time-consuming tasks. However, the price of our comfort has often resulted in more stress, overuse of stimulants, fragmentation of society, and a disconnection from nature and our real self. Ironically, there is less time to enjoy the comforts that the modern world brings. In these times of turbulence, there has been a surge in the popularity of yoga in the West.

In 1893, the first interest in yoga in the West was sparked by the discourses of Swami Vivekanada at the World Parliament of Religions in Chicago. Then followed the arrival of Paramahansa Yogananda on American soil in 1920, which resulted in thousands turning to the path of Kriya Yoga. In the 1960s, yoga philosophy was made fashionable by pop stars such as the Beatles, and charismatic yogis such as Bagwan Rajneesh, Shrila Prabhupada, and Maharishi Mahesh Yogi. Since then, the practice of yoga has grown steadily throughout the world, and has emerged as a mainstream form of exercise and a means of relieving stress caused by the demands of contemporary lifestyles.

Yoga's ability to integrate and accommodate all experiences and cultures can be likened to the subcontinent from which it emerged. Yoga has the ability to evolve, assimilate, and yet retain its essence. It has survived for thousands of years and will continue to affect and develop humanity.

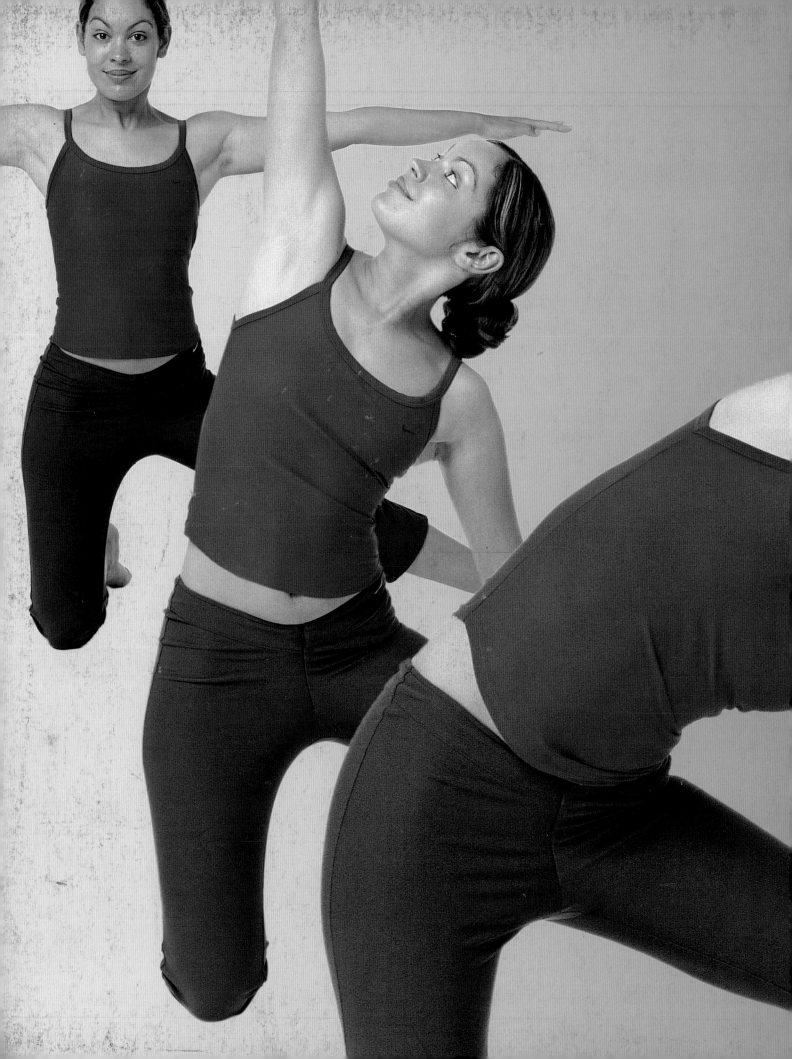

yoga, ancient and modern

Yoga is the art of proper action.
Bhagavad Gita

the story of yoga

yoga is...

several thousands of years old, and its survival and growth through the passage of time are a testament to its ascendancy. Its antiquity is revealed in the archaeological seals and scriptures of the Indus Valley, or Harappan, civilizations.

The ancient *rishis,* or seers, who renounced the world, studied and meditated to develop the system of yoga. In the course of their meditative practice they developed the yoga asanas through their observations of the movements of animals. At first, yoga teachings were passed from guru to disciple by word of mouth. In this way the clarity of meaning and purpose was maintained. One who follows the path of yoga is a yogi (male) or yogini (female).

the ancient scriptures

The philosophy of yoga is encapsulated in the ancient scriptures. They were written in Sanskrit, which is the oldest known language.

Veda means "knowledge" or "wisdom." Yoga is first mentioned in the vast collection of scriptures called the *Vedas,* which are believed to be *shruti,* or "divinely heard" mantras, revealed to ancient rishis in heightened meditative states. Veda Vyasa, a revered rishi, arranged the *Vedas* into four groups:

- *Rig-Veda,* "knowledge of hymns," is the oldest and is recited loudly.
- *Sama-Veda,* "knowledge of melodious chants," is the basis of Indian classical music.
- *Yajur-Veda,* "knowledge of sacrifice," is recited in a low voice.
- *Atharva-Veda* is "knowledge of mystical incantations."

The *Upanishads* are philosophical treatises that constitute the mystical part of the *Vedas* and provide the main foundation of yoga teaching. *Upanishad* is derived from *upa,* or "near," *ni,* or "down," and *shad,* or "to sit." Hence *Upanishad* means "sitting down near" and implies listening closely to the secret doctrines of a spiritual teacher. As the *Upanishads* form the concluding portion of the *Vedas,* they were called *Vedanta,* or "the end of *Vedas.*" They contain theories on the origins of the universe, the nature of the soul, and the connection between mind and matter.

In the last stages of Vedic literature, there emerged two epic poems. The *Ramayana,* written by the sage Valmiki, is an enthralling ethical poem written around the third century B.C. that gives a practical guidance on the Vedas through stories, expounding an ideal behavior and way of life. The *Mahabharata,* by Bhagavan Vyasa, is a comprehensive treatise on the science of society. It contains a poem called the *Bhagavad Gita,* which is probably the most noteworthy influence on yoga philosophy. *Bhagavad* means "divine one" and *gita* means "song." On the eve of a battle, the warrior Arjuna is suddenly struck with remorse at the thought of killing his kinsmen. The god Krishna instructs Arjuna that by carrying out his duty as a warrior, without attachment or malice, he will achieve liberation. Krishna conveys the meaning of yoga as "a deliverance from contact with pain and sorrow." The *Bhagavad Gita* describes three main paths of yoga:

- *Karma* yoga, or yoga of action, is wisdom in all action and work. Actions are carried out without thought of gain or praise, bringing mindfulness and knowledge of the self.
- *Jyana* yoga, or yoga of knowledge, is the yoga of the philosopher or thinker, and uses *buddhi,* or "intellect," to dismantle attachments, fears, sorrows, opinions, desires, hopes, and expectations to attain a deeper understanding of the true nature of the self.
- *Bhakti* yoga, or yoga of devotion, is the constant remembrance of the divine. Chanting, singing, dancing, and rituals are examples of Bhakti yoga.

the ancient texts

yoga sutra

The revered sage Patanjali systematized yoga philosophy some 2,000 years ago in the *Yoga Sutra* ("Aphorisms of Yoga"). The *Yoga Sutra* is credited as the classical text on *Raja* yoga, or royal yoga. Raja yoga is also called *Ashtanga* yoga. Ashtanga means "eight limbs."

The *Yoga Sutra* details 195 aphorisms divided into four *padas,* or chapters. The first chapter, called *samadhi pada,* describes the goal of meditation; the second and third define the eight limbs of Ashtanga yoga, which bring *samadhi* (see below). The last chapter details techniques for *moksha,* or "liberation."

The eight limbs of Ashtanga yoga are:

- *yama,* or abstinence—nonviolence, truthfulness, not stealing, continence, nonpossessiveness
- *niyama,* or observance—purity, contentment, austerity, self-study, dedication to god
- *asana,* or postures—steadiness, strength and suppleness, spinal flexibility
- *pranayama,* or breath control—preparing the mind for meditation
- *pratyahara,* or withdrawal of the senses—retracting the senses from the external world, focusing inward
- *dharana,* or concentration—fixing of the mind on a single point
- *dhyana,* or contemplation—complete absorption, without distraction, on an object
- *samadhi,* or absorption—absorption of consciousness into *brahman,* or superconsciousness

Hatha yoga, which constitutes *asana,* or postures, and *pranayama*, or breathing techniques, is a subdivision of Raja yoga. It is this type of yoga that this book will expound in detail in later sections. Most people in the West will begin with the practice of asanas. If the postures are practiced and mastered with integrity, grace, and balance, there will be a natural progression to practicing the other limbs of yoga.

yoga rahasya

The sage Nathamuni wrote *Yoga Rahasya* ("Secrets of Yoga") in the ninth century. The text gives detailed instructions on Ashtanga yoga and dictates that yoga practice for an individual should be carried out under the guidance of a teacher. *Yoga Rahasya* also gives guidance on the practice of yoga for pregnant women and as a way of treating illness and medical conditions.

hatha yoga pradipika

Swami Svatmarama wrote the *Hatha Yoga Pradipika* ("Light on Yoga") in Sanskrit. It describes techniques for asanas, pranayama, *mudra* (seals), *bandhas* (restraints), and internal cleansing practices, as well as the unblocking of the *nadis* (energy channels) and awakening of the *kundalini.* It is sometimes called *Sadanga* yoga, or "six-limb yoga." *Hatha Yoga Pradipika* advocates six cleansing *kriyas,* or "duties," to purify and prepare the physical body for asana practice. The six kriyas cleanse the digestive, eliminatory, and nervous systems. *Hatha Yoga Pradipika* has formed the basis of the modern practice of yoga.

gherunda samhita and siva samhita

These texts outline practices for the different paths of yoga that enable development of the higher self.

yogis of ancient times

shiva

Shiva is often attributed as being the original yogi and founder of yoga. He is often depicted as a dark-skinned ascetic sitting in the lotus position on a tiger skin, meditating at his abode in Mount Kailash. He is also shown riding on his bull, Nandi, carrying his trident. According to Hindu mythology, Shiva is the god of creation and destruction, which he enacts in Nataraja's dance. His creative role is symbolized by the frequently worshipped *lingam* (a stylized phallus worshiped as a symbol of the god Shiva).

matsyendra

In the *Hatha Yoga Pradipika,* Matsyendra, or "Lord of the Fishes," is reported to be one of the founders of Hatha yoga. He taught that, before embarking on the practices of meditation, the body and its elements need purifying. One of the asanas bears his name: Matsyendrasana (page 97).

patanjali

Patanjali is considered to be the "father of classical yoga." He is believed to be a teacher of yogic philosophy who, around the second century B.C., wrote the *Yoga Sutra* for his disciples who were training to be yoga teachers. Indeed, the *Yoga Sutra* continues to be studied and held in great merit by all serious students of yoga. In Indian mythology, he is considered to be an incarnation of the cosmic serpent Ananta, who serves the god Vishnu as an eternal couch.

shankaracharya

Shankaracharya was an Indian philosopher in the eighth century who founded *Advaita* (nondualistic) Vedanta. He left commentaries on the major Upanishads and advocated the indomitable search for logic and knowledge as a route to enlightenment.

yoga teachers of recent times

sri tirumalai krishnamacharya (1888–1989)

Krishnamacharya was born in Mysore, South India. His ancestry can be traced back to the famous ninth-century Indian sage Nathamuni. He studied the Vedic texts extensively from an early age with his father. At Banaras University, he studied Sanskrit, logic, and grammar. He also studied Vedanta and Samkhya, India's oldest philosophical system. In 1916 he met his teacher, Sri Ramamohan Brahmachari, at the foot of Mount Kailash. He spent more than seven years with this teacher, who gave him the great task of spreading the message of yoga and using his abilities to heal sick people. Hence, he studied Ayurveda, the traditional Indian healing system. In 1924, the Maharajah of Mysore, a devoted student, gave him the opportunity to open a yoga school in his palace. He finally settled in Madras with his wife and six children. Three notable students of Krishnamacharya's—T. K. V. Desikachar, B. K. S. Iyengar, and K. Pattabi Jois—developed his teachings and have become renowned teachers of yoga. His son, T. K. V. Desikachar, wrote *The Heart Of Yoga,* an inspirational book on developing personal practice. He advocates that the practice of yoga should be tailored to individuals' needs, to enable them to realize and fulfill their potential.

b. k. s. iyengar (born 1918)

B. K. S. Iyengar was born in 1918 in the village of Bellur, in Karnataka, India. In early childhood he had a variety of serious illnesses including malaria, tuberculosis, typhoid, and malnutrition. At the age of fifteen, he was invited to live with his sister by her husband, the great yoga teacher Sri Krishnamacharya. And so B.K.S. Iyengar began his training in yoga. Initially he struggled with the postures, but with determination and diligent practice he was able to improve. In 1937, he was instructed by his guru to go to Pune to teach yoga. Slowly, his recognition as a yoga teacher grew. In 1952, using yoga asanas, he remedied the frozen shoulder of violinist Yehudi Menuhin, who arranged for Mr. Iyengar to teach in London, Switzerland, and Paris. He is renowned for firmly establishing yoga in the West. With thousands of students in more than forty countries, he is probably the leading Hatha yoga master in the world today. He is the author of *Light on Yoga*, an indispensable book on Hatha yoga. At his center in Pune, his daughter Geeta, son Prashant, and senior teachers run regular classes.

k. pattabi jois (born 1915)

K. Pattabi Jois, born in 1915 in southern India, began his study of yoga under Sri Krishnamarchya at the age of twelve. Later he studied Sanskrit and Advaita philosophy at the Sanskrit college in Mysore. As a college professor, he taught Sanskrit and philosophy for thirty-six years. He began teaching yoga in 1937 and developed his style of yoga—Ashtanga yoga. This form of yoga is derived from *Yoga Korunta,* an ancient text written on leaves and bound together. Krishnamacharya and K. Pattabi Jois deciphered this ancient text, thought to be 5,000 years old. Hatha yoga is one of the eight limbs of Raja yoga, or Ashtanga yoga, and has long been recognized as the gateway to perfecting the other limbs. K. Pattabi Jois emphasizes the importance of achieving perfection in asana and pranayama as a path to attaining the other limbs outlined in Patanjali's *Yoga Sutra.* He describes perfection of the asana as being able to "sit for three hours with steadiness and happiness, with no trouble." From his home in Mysore, K. Pattabi Jois has instructed thousands of students from all over the world on this rigorous and purifying system of yoga.

paramahansa yogananda (1893–1952)

Paramahansa Yogananda was a truly great spiritual leader of the modern era. Swami Sivananda described him as "a rare gem of inestimable value, the like of whom the world has yet to witness." He is perhaps best known as the author of the inspiring spiritual classic, *Autobiography of a Yogi.* Paramahansa Yogananda was born in 1893 in Gorakhpur, India, near the Himalayas. At seventeen years of age, he began spiritual training under Swami Sri Yukteswar Giri, who instructed him in the path of Kriya yoga. He was conferred with the task of spreading the message of Kriya yoga to the West, to help unite the material power of the West with the spiritual power of the East.

swami sivananda (1887–1963)

Swami Sivananda is attributed with raising spiritual awareness in India and around the world. Born in the village of Pattamadai, southern India, he was named Kuppuswamy. He became a doctor and established a busy and thriving practice in Malaya, Malaysia. He still found time to study the scriptures and undertake yoga practice. In 1923, he renounced the world and began his pilgrimage around India. It eventually led him to Rishikesh. After years of intense and unbroken *sadhana,* he enjoyed the bliss of *nirvikalpa,* reaching the end of his spiritual journey. Swami Sivananda's yoga is known as the "yoga of synthesis," involving the harmonious development of the hand, head, and heart through the practice of Karma yoga, Jnana yoga, and Bhakti yoga. He founded the Divine Life Society in Rishikesh in 1936 and instituted the Sivananda Ayurvedic Pharmacy in 1945.

types of yoga

ananda yoga *Ananda* means "bliss" or "divine happiness." Swami Kriyananda, an American disciple of Paramahansa Yogananda, developed the techniques of Ananda yoga. The techniques involve use of silent affirmations interwoven with asanas and pranayama to control the subtle energies within oneself. Control of these energies helps to harmonize the body, mind, and emotions, awakening the greater power within.

anusara yoga *Anusara* means "following the heart" or "to step into the current of divine will." It was developed by John Friend and is described as heart-oriented, spiritually inspiring, and yet grounded in principles of precise body alignment. The three As of Anusara yoga are attitude, alignment, and action. Attitude refers to a pure spiritual expression of the heart when performing the asana. Alignment requires each asana to be performed with an integrated awareness of all the body parts. Action requires muscular and organic energy to hold the asana with stability. By following the three As, the mind, body, and spirit are equally honored.

bikram yoga Bikram yoga, developed by Bikram Choudhury, involves the practice of a series of twenty-six asanas in a well-heated room. The warm temperature, ranging between 80 and 100°F, is designed to warm and stretch the muscles, ligaments, and tendons to facilitate a deeper stretching of the muscles. The increased sweat detoxifies the body and the increase in heart rate yields a better cardiovascular workout. Bikram Choudhury studied yoga with Bishnu Ghosh, the brother of Paramahansa Yogananda. He teaches this style of yoga in his center in Beverly Hills.

integral yoga Swami Satchidananda, who was a student of Swami Sivananda, developed Integral yoga. He used the mantra "om" at the original Woodstock festival to raise the consciousness of thousands. Integral yoga places importance on using pranayama and meditation alongside asana practice. Dr. Dean Ornish uses Integral yoga to reverse the effects of heart disease.

iyengar yoga Iyengar yoga, named after B. K. S. Iyengar, emphasizes precise alignment, stability, firmness, and comfort when holding the asana. Props such as belts and blocks are used to assist this strive for perfection in the posture. By achieving exact alignment of the posture, maximum benefit is derived and energy is allowed to flow through the body. Iyengar teachers are required to complete two to five years of rigorous training for certification.

hatha yoga *Ha* means "sun" and *tha* means "moon." Hatha refers to the balance between the positive (sun) and the negative (moon) energies. It is one of the eight limbs of Patanjali's yoga and is probably the most widely practiced branch of yoga. Hatha yoga purifies the body to achieve perfect health and disciplines the mind in preparation for Raja yoga. It unlocks the individual's latent energies to enable self-development. Most contemporary styles of physical yoga emanate from Hatha yoga.

kali ray triyoga Kali Ray triyoga, founded by Kali Ray, combines posture, breath, and focus to create dynamic and intuitive flows. These flows involve synchronizing dynamic and sustained asana with the breath and mudra hand gestures. The triyoga flows are graded and adjusted according to ability.

kripalu yoga *Kripal* means "compassion" or "mercy." Kripalu yoga is called "the yoga of consciousness," and was founded by an Indian master named Kripalvananda. He was the spiritual teacher of yogi Amrit Desai, who took Kripalu yoga to America. Kripalu yoga places emphasis on body alignment and coordinating breath with movement. There are three stages to Kripalu yoga. First, yoga practice begins by exploring and aligning the body in a posture. Second, the student becomes attuned to the presence and flow of prana. In the third stage, there are spontaneous movements from one position to another, described as "meditation in motion."

kriya yoga *Kriya* means "action" or "rite." Kriya yoga is the ancient path of becoming self-realized by using techniques of energization, concentration, and meditation to gain awareness of the life process rather than the body. The breath, life energy, and consciousness are united to become one. Paramahansa Yogananda taught the scientific techniques of Kriya yoga to reach the highest states of divine consciousness and create a spiritual union with god—this is the underlying essence of all religions. The Self-Realization Fellowship, based in California and founded by Paramahansa Yogananda, teaches Kriya yoga techniques.

kundalini yoga *Kundalini* means "serpent power." In the physical body, kundalini resides at the base of the spine and, when awakened through yogic techniques, it rises up through the chakras (pages 24–25) until it reaches the chakra at the crown of the head, giving way to intuitive enlightenment. The breath of fire, a breathing technique where there is no separation between the inhalations and exhalations, *kriyas* (actions), and mantras are used to achieve kundalini awakening. The science of Kundalini yoga was kept secret for thousands of years until it was brought to the West by Yogi Bhajan in 1969. Once awakened, the latent kundalini energy is activated and a major change in consciousness is experienced.

sahaja yoga *Sahaja* means "spontaneous." In 1970, Sri Mataji Nirmala Devi introduced a simple and powerful method of meditation or inner awakening to bring spiritual ascent. The experience of the divinity is felt as a cool breeze over the crown of the head. As a result, physical, mental, and emotional balance is achieved and one becomes peaceful and joyous in life.

sivananda yoga The Sivananda system of yoga was developed by Swami Vishnu Devananda, who was sent to the West by his teacher, Sivananda, to draw people onto the yogic path. It is one of the largest schools of yoga. Sivananda yoga advocates practicing five principles: classic asana practice, pranayama, meditation, relaxation, and a proper diet. Swami Devananda has established an international network of Sivananda yoga centers.

svaroopa yoga Svaroopa yoga was developed by Rama Berch. He promotes a different emphasis during asana practice. At first the focal point is the base of the spine, progressing upward through each spinal area. The aim is to develop the transcendent inner experience and thereby raise consciousness.

tantric yoga *Tantra* means "where opposites unite" and is symbolized in uniting the female and masculine forces, shiva and shakti. It is often misinterpreted as involving sexual union. The teachings of Tantric yoga are well guarded and should be learned only from a master.

viniyoga Viniyoga was first taught by Krishnamacharya, who emphasized fluidity in movement from one asana to another and the use of the breath to coordinate the movement. In Viniyoga practice, postures are selected to suit the individual's abilities.

vinyasa ashtanga yoga *Vinyasa* means "breath-synchronized movement" and *Ashtanga* means "eight limbs." Vinyasa Ashtanga yoga practice involves moving gracefully through a continual dynamic flow of specific asanas synchronized with breathing techniques. Ujjayi breathing (page 29) is used to generate internal body heat. This, combined with two important internal *bandhas,* or body locks, induces profuse sweating during the sequence, which eliminates toxins. There is a dramatic increase in energy and well-being. Circulation is enhanced and flexibility, strength, stamina, balance, and concentration are maximized. This system, developed by K. Pattabi Jois, is not for beginners and should be undertaken only under the guidance of a teacher. In the West, so-called power yoga is based on Ashtanga yoga.

yoga and healthy eating

The practice of yoga invariably leads to a greater awareness of nutrition. Ayurveda, a system of healing thought to be 5,000 years old, evolved on the Indian subcontinent, around the same time as yoga. It uses herbs and exercise, massage, meditation, and the correct nutrition to achieve a healthy and well-balanced body. The science of Ayurveda classifies food according to three types of *gunas*, or "energies":

• Rajasic food is very hot, bitter, sour, salty, or dry. Examples include chilies, chutney, pickles, tea, coffee, eggs, and chocolate. A yogic diet should limit or exclude the intake of rajasic foods because they overstimulate the mind and body, excite the passions, and cause mental stress and restlessness.

• Tamasic food is overcooked or processed food, which reduces the flow of prana energy through the body and produces lethargy and feelings of despondency. Examples of tamasic food include fish, meat, alcohol, tobacco, onions, and garlic. A diet high in tamasic food lowers the body's resistance to disease.

• Sattvic food is a pure, wholesome diet of foods such as wholegrain bread, fresh fruit juices, fresh or dried fruit, seeds, nuts, honey, milk, and butter. These are foods identified as being high in vital vitamins and minerals. They are also the foods that are most easily digested. A diet high in sattvic food maintains the homeostasis of the body, calms and purifies the mind, and increases energy levels. It is the diet that is the most suitable for the serious yoga practitioner.

rajasic food   tamasic food   sattvic food

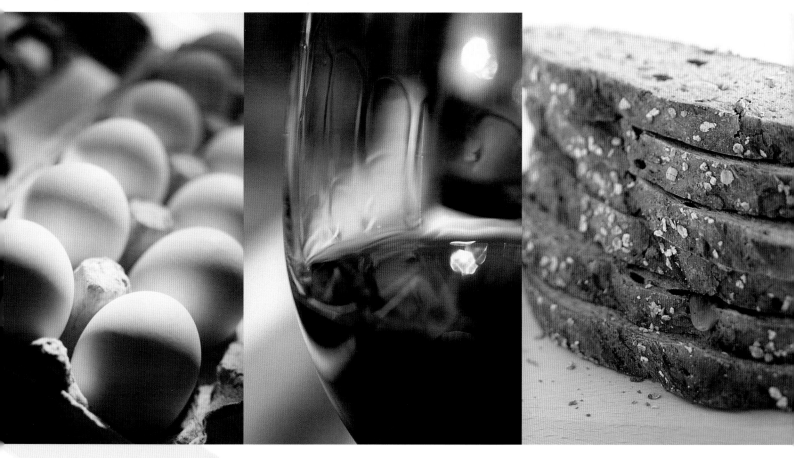

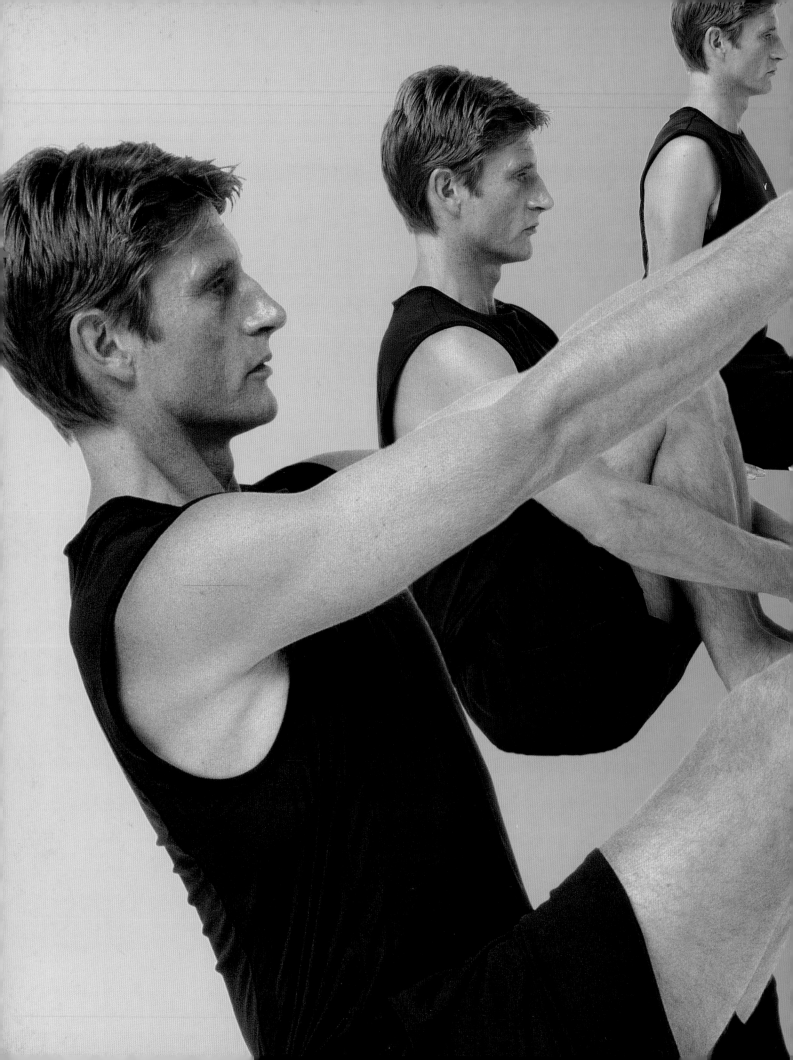

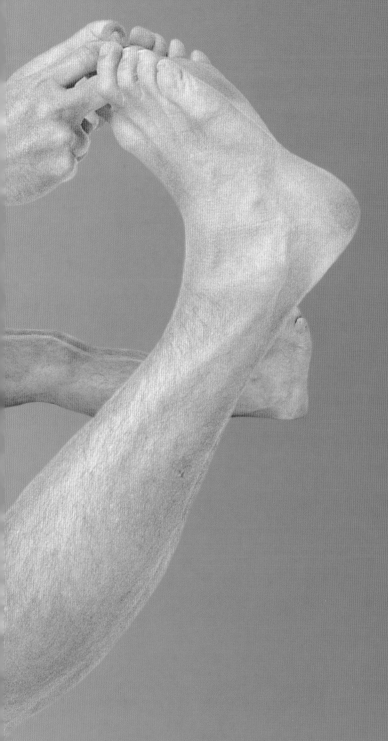

learning the
postures

preparation for yoga

where should I practice?
Before beginning, prepare the environment. A quiet, clean, and clutter-free room is ideal. The room should be warm and well-ventilated, and with enough floor space to lie stretched out. Ideally the floor space should be about eight square feet for people of average height and nine square feet for tall individuals.

do I need special clothes?
Wear comfortable clothes that are not tight, particularly around the waist. If it is warm, then keep clothes to a minimum. The feet should be bare and all jewelry should be removed. You may want to have a shawl or blanket on hand to cover the body when lying in Savasana (page 91).

what do I need to practice?
Yoga should preferably be practiced on a nonslip surface such as a yoga mat or a rug. Most sporting outlets and yoga centers now sell yoga mats. Sitting asanas for meditation can be carried out on a cushion and wool blanket. Teachers of Western audiences have devised a variety of equipment that can be used to aid positioning in the posture. Using equipment such as wooden blocks, wedges, and ropes is a personal preference. It is certainly not a necessity. Yoga can be practiced anywhere without having to lug equipment around.

when should I practice?
Early mornings and evenings are usually good times to practice. In the mornings the body is fresh and energetic, but can be stiff. Hence the morning routine should incorporate postures to gently stretch out the body's stiffness. Many teachers advocate doing yoga every morning for a few minutes to allow the body to be energized and the mind to remain alert through the day. In the evenings, the body may be tired but with less joint and muscle stiffness. The evening routine should incorporate postures to rejuvenate the body. Alternatively, if carried out before bedtime, stretches conducive to sleep can be practiced. Asanas, unless specified otherwise, should be practiced two hours after a heavy meal and one hour after a light meal.

how often do I practice?
The frequency of practice is a personal choice. Initially, set a regular time to practice once a week. Often there is a natural progression to increasing the length and frequency of practice. Ideally, yoga should be practiced at least three times a week to accrue benefits. Regular practice is important in establishing yoga as a discipline and developing awareness of the mind and body.

the hatha yoga asanas A large variety of asanas are illustrated in this book, offering a wide experience of yoga. Also shown are key body positions (or setting up postures) that lead into the asana with comprehensive step-by-step instructions. For example, on page 39, Tadasana, or Mountain posture, represents the starting position for many of the standing asanas in this section. On each asana, there is a brief introductory note with the particular benefits to be gained in practice. Where necessary, cautions have been given.

guidelines and cautions for practice

guidelines

• Always prepare the muscles with warm-up exercises before practicing yoga postures. This not only assists in attaining the correct position and sustaining the position but also prevents muscle cramps or other injuries.

• Move slowly and gently in and out of the postures. Focus the mind on the posture and don't rush from one posture to another.

• Be attentive to the specific body positions needed to attain the posture. Work to a level that is comfortable for the body. If a posture is difficult to achieve, then do not overstretch the spine or muscles to achieve the position. Instead, practice an easier variation or another posture that is more comfortable and gives similar benefits. After a few weeks, try the difficult posture again.

• Once the correct position has been attained, let the breath steadily flow in and out through the nostrils. The eyes should have a soft focus or be closed to enable an inward focus.

cautions

• If pain or discomfort is experienced when holding a posture, consult a yoga therapist who can advise on counterstretches. Frequent practice of the counterstretch can eliminate the discomfort or pain experienced in the posture. If pain continues to persist, then seek medical advice.

• In some of the postures, the flow of blood is reversed. If this causes light-headedness or dizziness, then gently release from the posture and adopt one of the relaxed postures; for example: Balasana (see page 56) or Sarvangasana (see page 117).

• Individuals with high blood pressure and heart problems should avoid standing poses, inversions, and the strenuous backward and forward bends. Also avoid jumping when practicing standing positions with feet wide apart. If in any doubt, seek medical advice.

• The Sun salutation and inversions are not recommended for women during menstruation.

• During pregnancy, yoga should be practiced under the guidance of an antenatal yoga teacher. In general, the following should be avoided: Sun salutation, standing postures during the first three months, inversions, prone postures, forward bends, and backward bends. Many of the postures can be carried out but in an adapted form, which avoids pressure on the abdomen.

variations Yoga is adaptable to each individual's needs and hence there are many variations to each asana. These can be used when an asana is difficult to attain and an easier body position is needed, or when the asana has been mastered and a further stretch is even more beneficial. A variation shown at the same level enables exploration of the asana. Variations of an asana are clearly identified within a box, and labeled according to the level of ability, e.g., beginner or intermediate.

physiology

muscles

Muscle is principally made up of fibrous and connective tissue, both of which contribute to its elasticity. The muscles in the body are arranged in layers so that movement can be carried out through contrasting muscle forces. For example, when the elbow is flexed, the arm flexors contract to pull while the arm extensor is reciprocally relaxed. The muscle activating the movement is the agonist; the muscle controlling the speed and extent of movement is the antagonist. The agonists are shortened, while the antagonists are relaxed to help sustain the movement. The science of yoga has been designed to give all muscles the opportunity to act as agonist or antagonist. The asanas give muscles a slow, gentle stretch. As the breath is deepened, the supply of oxygen and blood flow to the muscles is increased to boost strength and elasticity. The accumulation of lactic acid in the muscles is prevented and circulation to the tissues and organs is enhanced. Elasticity of the muscles aids greater joint mobility and spinal flexibility.

skeleton

The skeletal frame is arranged symmetrically, making up an intricate framework of 206 bones. The vertebral column is composed of thirty-three bones, separated by intervertebral discs and grouped as shown below:

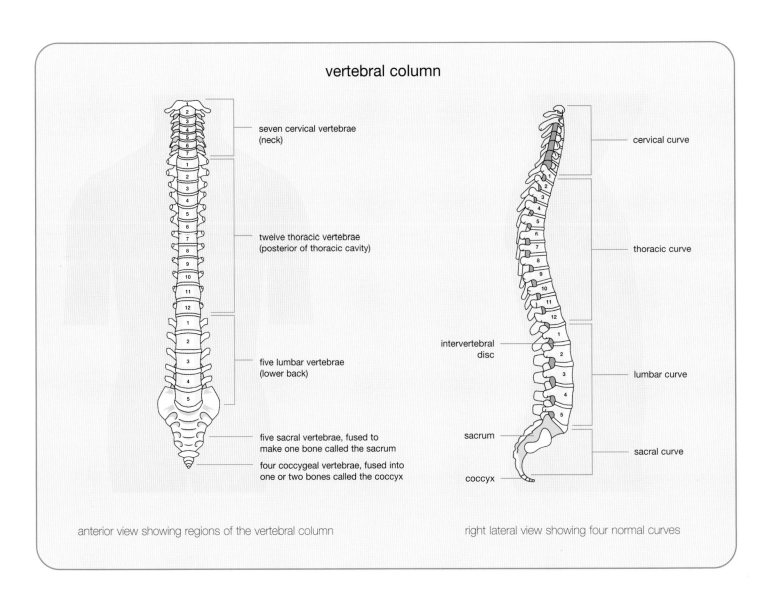

vertebral column

seven cervical vertebrae
(neck)

twelve thoracic vertebrae
(posterior of thoracic cavity)

five lumbar vertebrae
(lower back)

five sacral vertebrae, fused to
make one bone called the sacrum

four coccygeal vertebrae, fused into
one or two bones called the coccyx

cervical curve

thoracic curve

intervertebral
disc

lumbar curve

sacrum

sacral curve

coccyx

anterior view showing regions of the vertebral column

right lateral view showing four normal curves

spine

The spine is the central axis of the body and combines with the joints and muscles to make a supportive frame for the trunk to maintain an upright posture. The movements of the thorax enable the ventilation of the lungs. The trunk holds and protects the internal organs such as the liver and kidneys. The spinal cord is protectively enclosed inside the vertebral column.

Infants have very flexible spines and they actively utilize the full range of movement available. However, over the course of years there is a tendency to lose that flexibility. Our lifestyles often give rise to poor posture, rounded shoulders, and a hollow back, which can increase the possibility of lower back pain and poor breathing patterns. The yoga asanas work on flexing and extending different sections of the spine and regaining the range of movements available to the spinal column. The mobility between the intervertebral disks is increased and the spine is strengthened, with increased flexibility. The body's energy is said to flow along paths linking the chakras, which are aligned along the spinal column (pages 24–25). By keeping the spine flexible, the flow of energy is enabled to run smoothly along the *sushumna,* or spinal energy channel. Thus energy levels throughout the day are improved.

the spine in the asanas

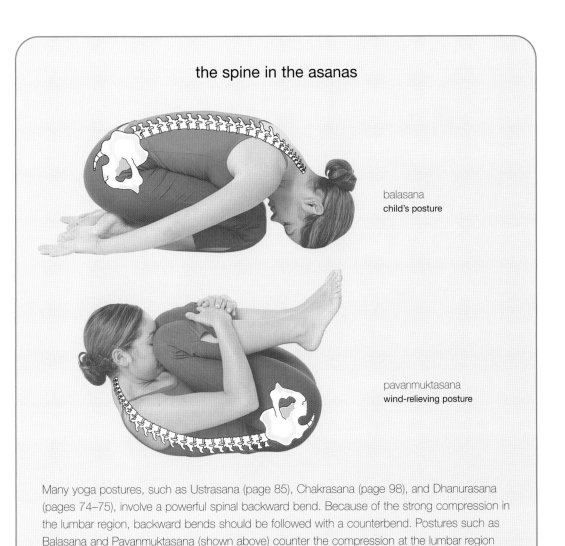

balasana
child's posture

pavanmuktasana
wind-relieving posture

Many yoga postures, such as Ustrasana (page 85), Chakrasana (page 98), and Dhanurasana (pages 74–75), involve a powerful spinal backward bend. Because of the strong compression in the lumbar region, backward bends should be followed with a counterbend. Postures such as Balasana and Pavanmuktasana (shown above) counter the compression at the lumbar region and stretch the flexor muscles involved in the backward bend.

nadis, chakras & the subtle body

The "subtle breath" prana flows through the *nadis,* or energy channels, in the "subtle body" that are connected to the seven *chakras,* or energy centers. *Chakra,* which means "wheel," is a vortex of pranic energy that equates to the body's nerve plexus. The central nadi runs through the center of the spinal column. This is known as *sushumna.* Running along either side of the sushumna are two important nadis, *ida* and *pingala,* which lead to the openings of the nostrils. Six of the chakras are aligned along the sushumna, while the seventh is located at the crown of the head.

The practice of Hatha yoga, pranayama, and meditation is concerned with balancing out or purifying the flows in the nadis at all levels by eliminating physical, emotional, and psychic blockages. By activating the chakras, a higher level of awareness and consciousness is experienced. Visualization of the colors and mantras that correspond to the chakras is a more intense and concentrated way of attuning and harmonizing the flow of prana through the nadis and chakras.

At the base of the spine in the muladhara chakra lies the dormant *kundalini,* or "serpent power," which is said to be a concentration of cosmic life energy. When the kundalini is awakened, it travels upward along the spine to the sahasrara chakra at the crown of the head. Awakening the kundalini by yogic practices enables conscious awareness of the presence of the cosmic power within us. The practice of awakening this dormant power should be carried out only under the guidance of an experienced teacher or guru.

The seven chakras are as follows:

	muladhara chakra	swadhishthana chakra	manipura chakra	anahata chakra	vishddha chakra rishuddha	ajna chakra	sahasrara chakra
translation	root-prop wheel	own-base wheel	jewel-city wheel	wheel of the unstuck sound	wheel of purity	command wheel	thousand-spoked petal
visual form	a lotus of four petals	a lotus of six petals	a lotus of ten petals	a lotus of twelve petals	a lotus of sixteen petals	a lotus of two petals	a lotus of 1,000 petals
location	base of spine	genitals	navel	heart	throat	between eyebrows	crown of head
plexus	pelvic plexus	sacral plexus	solar plexus	cardiac plexus	laryngeal plexus	associated with the mind	associated with the brahman or superconscious
vital activity	sense of smell	sense of taste	sense of sight	sense of touch	sense of hearing	mental activity	
element	earth	water	fire	air	ether		
color	yellow	light blue	red	smoky green	purple	snow-white	many colors
mantra	lam	vam	ram	yam	ham	om (aum)	visarga
shape	square	circle	triangle	hexagram	crescent	white circle with two petals	formless
ruling body	Mars	Mercury	Sun	Venus	Jupiter	Saturn	

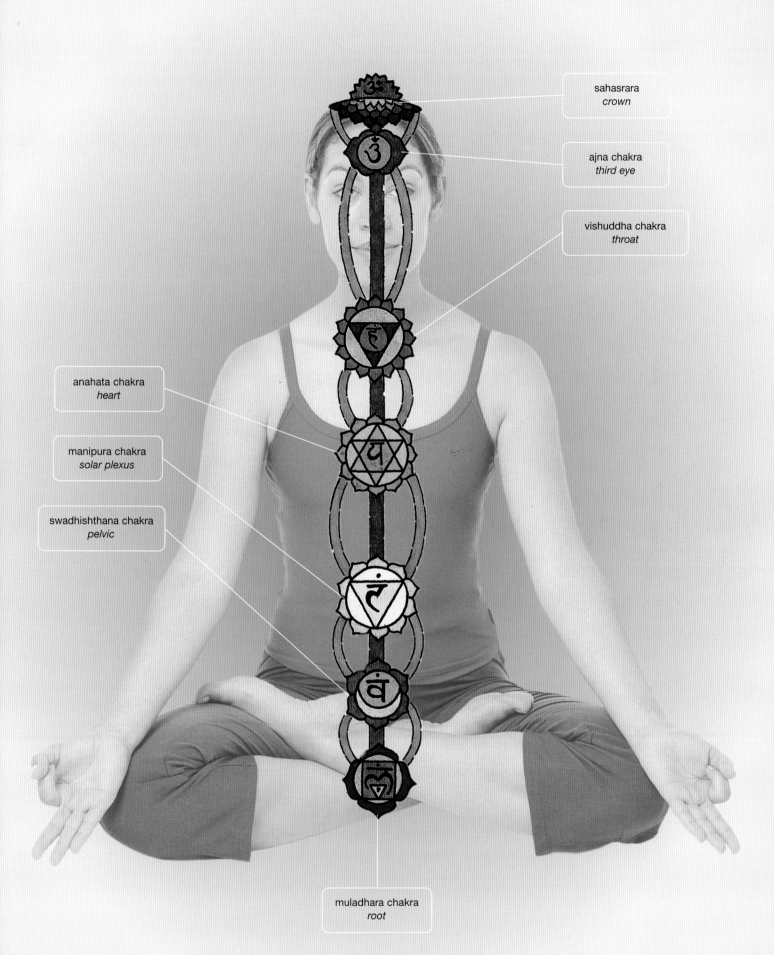

sahasrara
crown

ajna chakra
third eye

vishuddha chakra
throat

anahata chakra
heart

manipura chakra
solar plexus

swadhishthana chakra
pelvic

muladhara chakra
root

prana

Pra means "first" and *na* means "unit." Prana is the subtle universal energy that pervades all entities. Prana exists in living and nonliving matter. Heat, light, gravity, electricity, magnetism, etc. are all forms of prana. It is the reason that Earth follows its orbital path around the Sun and the rivers flow toward the ocean, which surges under the radiance of the Moon. It is the reason that there is life on Earth. For living entities, prana is the vital energy or the life force that flows continuously through the body. Breathing is a prominent manifestation of prana. *Chitta,* which means "consciousness," is closely interlinked with prana. When the breath is steady and even, the mind and prana vibrations are also steady and even. It was from this realization that the ancient yogis devised the practice of pranayama.

pranayama

what is pranayama? *Prana* refers to the breath and *ayama* means "stretch" or "extend." Pranayama is the fourth of the eight limbs of yoga. Pranayama is the control, harmonization, and integration of prana through the regulation of the breath.

what are the stages of pranayama? Pranayama emphasizes control in the inhalation, exhalation, and suspension of the breath. The stages of pranayama are as follows:

• *Puraka,* or inhalation, should be smooth and even. At this stage, the air is allowed to flow in freely by expanding the chest and drawing the ribs outward and upward.

• *Antara kumbhaka,* or "internal breath retention," is when the air is held in the lungs. The retention of the breath is important and used in some pranayama techniques, but it should not be forced and should be practiced only when it does not interfere with the fluidity of a full inhalation and exhalation.

• *Rechaka,* or "exhalation," in pranayama techniques requires the complete expulsion of the air from the lungs. The control and regulation of the exhalation are vital as the impurities are eliminated at this stage; this increases the lung's capacity for the new breath to penetrate deep into the body. Generally speaking, rechaka should last longer than puraka.

• *Bhaya kumbhaka,* or "external breath retention," is when the lungs are held empty. This technique is generally carried out only at an advanced level.

what techniques are used to control the breathing stages? *Bandhas,* or "locks," are specific postures in which certain muscles are tensed to intensify stages of pranayama. The bandhas should be used only by experienced practitioners and under the guidance of a teacher. The Jalandhara bandha or "chin pressing against the breast bone" position is used to obstruct the airway and keep air from escaping. Uddhiyana bandha, or "full retraction of the abdomen," is used at the end of rechaka and during bhaya kumbhaka so that air is prevented from entering the lungs. Muladhara bandha involves contracting the anal sphincter muscles and is used during the kumbhaka stages when air is either retained or prevented from entering the lungs. The bandhas should be released gently when progressing to inhaling or exhaling.

what are the benefits? Pranayama requires minimal physical exertion, but is able to increase oxygen intake considerably. The increased oxygen flow permeates deep into every cell of the body. Hence, pranayama is said to regenerate the body's cells, enhance well-being, and aid healing. The breath is said to be the bridge between the mind and the body, and between the conscious and unconscious. By focusing on the breath, the mind becomes calm and integrated.

does it improve health? Stress, anxiety, poor posture, and exposure to air pollutants can cause shallow breathing and reduce the flow of prana in the body. Ill health is said to arise when the nadis and chakras are blocked. The practice of asanas and pranayama is designed to unblock the energy pathways and let the energy flow smoothly along the spine.

does it increase life span? The longevity of the body is said to increase as the number of breaths taken is reduced (but with increased efficiency). Many yogis are reputed to exceed a hundred years of age by the practice of pranayama. In the animal world, there is a strong correlation between the number of breaths and the life span. For example the giant tortoise, which takes three breaths in a minute, can live over 180 years, whereas a monkey, which takes thirty breaths a minute, has a life span of about twenty to thirty years.

when is the optimum time to practice? Pranayama should be carried out after the asanas. It is the natural progression from asana practice. Always finish the asana practice with Savasana (page 91), before practicing pranayama. The duration of practice should initially be about three minutes and gradually build to twenty minutes. Early morning is the optimum time for practice, but if this is not possible, then practicing at any part of the day will also yield benefits.

can beginners practice pranayama? Pranayama should at first be practiced under the guidance of a good yoga teacher. The teacher will determine when to begin practice and what techniques are suitable.

which positions are suitable for pranayama practice? Pranayama can be carried out in any sitting position that is comfortable and enables the spine to be held erect. If the spine cannot be held erect, then begin by lying in supine position. The head should be held level and centered. Ensure that clothing does not restrict the movement of the rib cage and diaphragm. The hands can either be cupped together on the lap or held in the jnana mudra (page 33).

Positions for Pranayama:

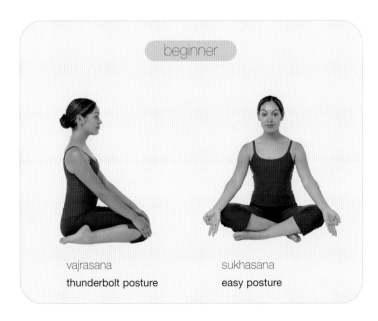

beginner

vajrasana
thunderbolt posture

sukhasana
easy posture

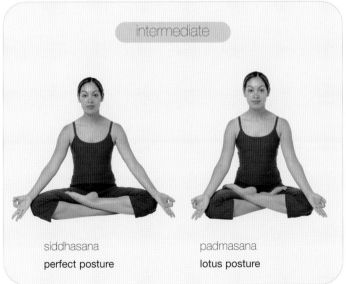

intermediate

siddhasana
perfect posture

padmasana
lotus posture

pranayama techniques

kapalabhati, cleansing breath

Kapala means "skull" and *bhati* means "that which brings lightness." Kapalabhati is a cleansing pranayama technique for eliminating stale air in the lungs. It is also one of the six kriyas, or cleansing practices. This invigorating practice is a useful way of beginning pranayama. In this technique the breath is deliberately performed faster. The abdomen and diaphragm act as a pump during the exhalations.

level: Beginner/Intermediate

benefits: • Increases intake of oxygen • Brings clarity to the mind • Improves concentration and focus

❶ Breathe normally, focusing on the breath. Then, on the exhalation, contract the abdominal muscles sharply, pushing up the diaphragm and expelling all the air with speed through the nostrils, making a sighing sound.

❷ Relax the abdominal muscles and inhale. The inhalation is passive and silent. The inhalation period is longer than the exhalation period. Repeat for ten to twenty breaths, maintaining a forceful exhalation.

❸ Inhale and exhale normally once. On the next inhalation, retain the breath for as long as it is comfortable. Slowly exhale and return to normal breathing. Observe the effect on the mind.

anuloma viloma, alternate nostril breathing

Anuloma means "with the hair" or "with order," and *viloma* means "against the hair" or "against order." *Anuloma viloma* is also known as the "sun and moon breath," as it harmonizes the masculine (sun) and feminine (moon) energies. It is another gentle cleansing technique. The dominant hand adopts the Vishnu mudra: the index and middle finger are pressed into the palm while the thumb acts with the ring and little finger to open and close the nostrils alternately.

level: Beginner

benefits: • Purifies the nadis • Soothes the nervous system • Calms the mind

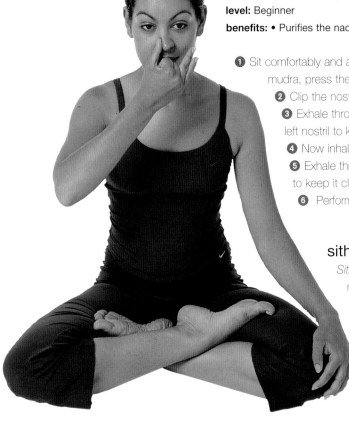

❶ Sit comfortably and adopt the Vishnu mudra. Assuming the right hand is used to form the mudra, press the thumb against the right nostril and inhale through the left nostril.

❷ Clip the nostrils together to retain the breath.

❸ Exhale through the right nostril while pressing the ring and little finger against the left nostril to keep it closed.

❹ Now inhale through the right nostril, still keeping the left one closed.

❺ Exhale through the left nostril while pressing the thumb against the right nostril to keep it closed.

❻ Perform three to five rounds of the cycle. Gradually increase to twenty.

sithali, cooling breath

Sithali means "cool." This technique is unusual because the inhalation is made through the mouth, whereas the exhalation is through the nostrils. The tongue is rolled up to make a channel. If this is not possible, then perform a similar technique called Sitkari, where the inhalation is through a small gap between the lips and teeth, and exhalation through the nostrils.

level: Intermediate

benefits: • Purifies the blood • Quenches thirst • Stimulates the liver and spleen

❶ Draw the tongue out and curl the sides up to make a channel. The tip of the tongue protrudes out slightly. Inhale slowly through this channel, as if sipping air through a straw.

❷ Close the mouth as the breath is retained for a few seconds. Press the tongue against the palate.

❸ Exhale slowly through the nostrils. Repeat for five cycles.

brahmari, bee breath

Brahmari means "bee." In this breathing exercise, the inhalation sound is akin to the humming of a male bee, whereas the exhalation sound is likened to the humming of a female bee.

level: Intermediate

benefits: • Calms the mind • Beneficial for pregnant women preparing for labor • Improves the quality of the voice

❶ Partially close the glottis (by contracting the upper end of the windpipe) and inhale through both the nostrils with force.

❷ Exhale slowly through both nostrils. The inhalation and exhalation should be smooth so that a continuous and even sound is produced. Repeat the cycle five to ten times.

❸ To enhance the humming sounds, press the thumbs against the ears.

ujjayi, victorious breath

Jaya means "victory" or "conquest." In this technique, the emphasis is on fully expanding the chest.

level: Intermediate/Advanced

benefits: • Strengthens the nervous system • Relieves tiredness • Removes excess phlegm, gas, or bile

❶ Breathe through both nostrils. Begin with a deep exhalation and expand the chest for a deep inhalation.

❷ Contract the larynx (located at the back of the throat) to narrow the air passage slightly. Feel the passage of air resonating at the back of the throat to produce a faint snore. Compress the abdomen gently to expel as much air as possible. Observe the rhythmic movements of the chest and ribs. Repeat five times.

❸ For the next stage, inhale and exhale as above, but retain the breath for two to three seconds. In advanced practice, the Jalandhara and Muladhara bandhas can be applied to lengthen the duration of Antara kumbhaka. Repeat for five cycles.

manipura, breathing

Manipura means "jewel-city." Manipura breathing is sometimes known as "the breath of fire." The manipura chakra is located at the navel and corresponds to the solar plexus. This technique involves directing prana to a specific area of the body. It develops the ability to direct prana to other parts of the body, e.g., for increasing warmth to the extremities.

level: Intermediate/Advanced

benefits: • Cleanses the lungs • Improves circulation • Brings clarity to the mind • Increases energy levels

❶ Take deep breaths through the nostrils, focusing deeply on the breath for one to two minutes.

❷ On the exhalation, contract the navel inward toward the spine.

❸ On the inhalation, relax the muscles around the navel, and through concentrated focus, draw the pranic energy of the breath deep into the navel.

❹ Repeat the cycle five to ten times.

meditation

In our waking consciousness, the mind is preoccupied with absorbing external stimuli and wandering from one thought to another. Yoga meditation turns this outward perspective inward to seek the inner sanctum of silence, peace, and harmony. The clamor of rapid thoughts, of the past, present, and future, are reduced and the mind is quieted. Stilling the mind enables mental clarity and poise. Patanjali describes meditation as a combination of three steps:

1. *Pratyahara,* or withdrawal of the senses
2. *Dharana,* or concentration
3. *Dhyana,* or contemplation

Meditation can be carried out in Sukhasana (page 27) or Ardha padmasana (page 63) or Padmasana (page 63). The hands can either be placed on the lap with palms facing upward, or the jnana mudra adopted (page 33). Sit facing east with the spine erect. Begin by allowing the mind to become absorbed in the sound of the rhythmic breath flowing in and out. The ideal time to practice is in the morning after waking or in the evening. There are many techniques of meditation; some simple techniques are described here.

breathing meditation

This technique develops pratyahara, or sense withdrawals, and involves the conscious experience of prana.

❶ Sit comfortably, gradually absorbing the mind in the breath. Simply by observing the breath, the inhalation and exhalation will be deepened. Feel the coolness deep inside the head when inhaling and the warmth inside the lower nostrils while exhaling.

❷ Mentally repeat "shanti" (peace) when inhaling, and "mukti" (freedom) when exhaling. Other similar phrases can be used such as "peace is my real nature" and "not conflict" when exhaling. Continue for two to three minutes at first, building up to ten minutes.

candle meditation

Candle meditation is a type of *trataka,* or "steady gazing," and is one of the six purifying processes of Hatha yoga. It involves focusing on one image to develop dharana, or concentration.

❶ Sit comfortably in a darkened room with a candle flame at eye level. Place the candle about three feet away. Fix the gaze on the candle flame. Avoid blinking.

❷ Close the eyes. When they become watery, visualize the image of the candle at the Ajna or Anahata chakra (pages 24–25). When the internal candle image dissipates, open the eyes and repeat gazing at the candle. Initially the attention may slip away and thoughts may intrude. Let the mind wander for a while and then return to the focal point of the candle and continue. The aim is to increase the time spent gazing at the candle with eyes open.

japa or repetition of mantra

Mantras are Sanskrit syllables or words, which are considered to be powerful sounds that enable the conscious and unconscious to merge. By the continuous repetition of a mantra for several minutes, the pulsating flow of thoughts is stemmed and mental energy is directed toward a higher consciousness. Mantras develop dharana, or concentration. If carried out with a deeper spiritual focus, then dhyana, or contemplation, is also developed. Ideally, only one mantra should be used during meditative practice to accustom the mind to its sound patterns. Short mantras should be used at first. A teacher or guru can select a suitable mantra for an individual. Alternatively, try out some mantras yourself and select the one that brings a sense of harmony. Mantras can be repeated either silently or aloud. The latter is preferred, however, as the sound will resonate internally. For mantras to be effective, they need to be pronounced clearly. A small selection of mantras is given here. Each chakra, or energy center, has a mantra associated with it, which can also be used (pages 24–25).

mantras

- *Om* (aum) means "infinite spirit." This sound resonates as a perfect circle and is the root of all sounds and letters. The "o" sound begins deep within the body with lips slightly apart and is slowly drawn upward joining with the "m" sound, which is carried out with lips together and resonates through the entire head.
- *Om shanti shanti shanti* is said to bring harmony. *Shanti* means "peace" and is repeated three times. The duration of the "Om" sound is shorter.
- *Hari om tat sat* means "the lord is the infinite spirit." The hari is said as "ha-ri," and "om" is described above. *Tat* and *sat* are said without lingering on the sound.
- *Soham* (soh-hum) means "I am that." This mantra is repeated with the inhalation ("so") and exhalation ("ham"). The sound "soham" resembles the reverberating, natural sound of breathing.

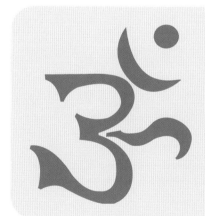

om "Om" is a mantra or prayer in itself. Although "om" symbolizes the most profound concepts of Hindu belief, it is in use daily. The Hindus begin their day or any work or a journey by uttering "om." The sacred symbol is often found at the head of letters, at the beginning of examination papers, and so on. Many Hindus, as an expression of spiritual perfection, wear the sign of "om" as a pendant. This symbol is enshrined in every Hindu temple or in some form or another on family shrines.

hasta mudras (hand gestures)

Hasta means "hand," and *mudra* means "closing" or "sealing." Hasta mudras are gestures of the hands, embodying specific positions of the fingers, wrist, and palms. The ancient yogis mapped out the position of meridians, or nadis, on the hand areas. They are an important part of meditation and have a therapeutic effect on the mind and body. By joining, folding, or bending the fingers and palms, the meridians are activated or unblocked and balance is achieved. Each finger is represented by one of the five universal elements and is connected to one of the body's energy centers, or chakras (pages 24–25).

❶ *angustha,* or "thumb"
　　represents *agni,* or "fire element"
　　linked to manipura chakra, or "solar plexus"

❷ *tarjani,* or "index finger"
　　represents *vayu,* or "air element"
　　linked to anahata chakra, or "cardiac plexus"

❸ *madhyama,* or "middle finger"
　　represents *akash,* or "ether element"
　　linked to vishuddha chakra, or "laryngeal plexus"

❹ *anamika,* or "ring finger"
　　represents *prithvi,* or "earth element"
　　linked to muladhara chakra, or "pelvic plexus"

❺ *kanishthika,* or "little finger"
　　represents *jal,* or "water element"
　　linked to swadhishthana chakra, or "sacral plexus"

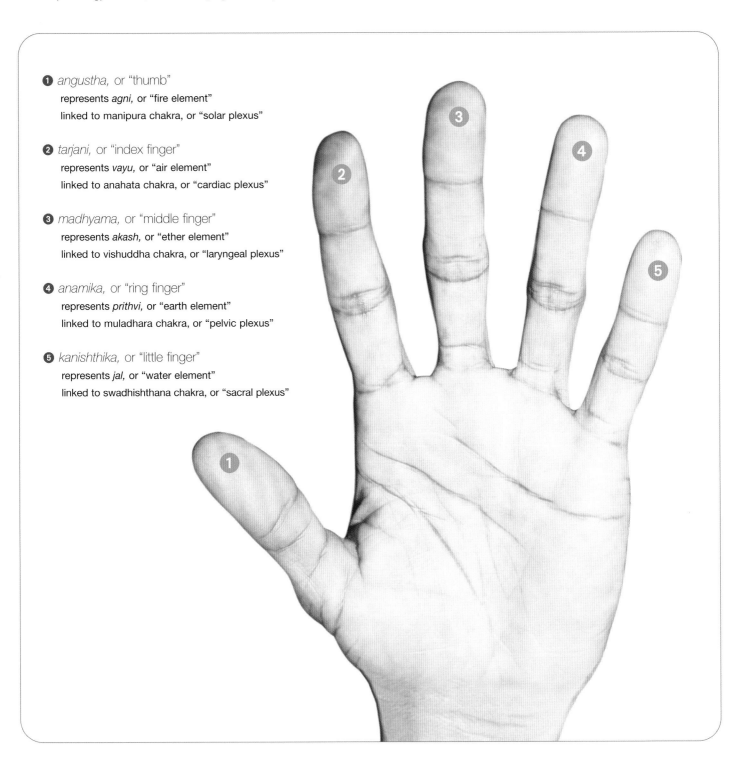

There are thousands of hasta mudras. A few of the popular mudras are illustrated below:

linga mudra

benefits: • Increases warmth of the body • Reduces coughs • Eliminates constipation

Clasp the fingers of both hands firmly and raise the inner thumb erect and point away from the other fingers.

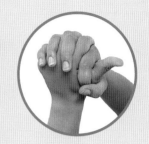

jnana mudra

benefits: • Enables concentration when meditating • Bestows memory and intelligence • Brings calmness and serenity

Join the tips of the index finger and thumb. The remaining three fingers are kept straight.
Used for meditation, this mudra can be held for the duration of the meditation.

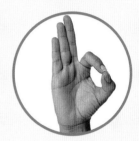

shunya mudra

benefits: • Improves hearing • Alleviates ear disorders • Promotes patience

Bend the longest middle finger and press the nail against the soft part of the thumb.
To gain benefits, this mudra needs to be carried out daily for a few minutes.

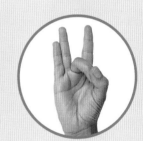

surya mudra

benefits: • Reduces excess fat in the body • Revitalizes the nervous system • Promotes creativity

Bend the ring finger and press the flesh under the nail against the soft part of the thumb.

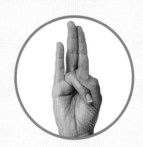

prana mudra

benefits: • Increases pranic energy • Promotes better health • Improves weak eyesight

Join the tips of the ring and little finger with that of the thumb. The remaining two fingers are kept straight. This mudra can be performed for any length of time.

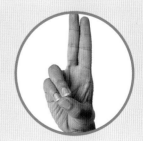

warming up

For the beginner or intermediate practitioner of yoga, it is advisable to spend a few minutes warming up. Warm-up stretches prepare the muscles and joints for the yoga asanas and reduce the risk of muscle strain, cramps, or other injuries. They also help to position the body in the asana and to sustain the position for longer. When planning a warm-up routine, select exercises that will stretch all parts of the body. Exercises can be selected from those shown below, but many others can be used.

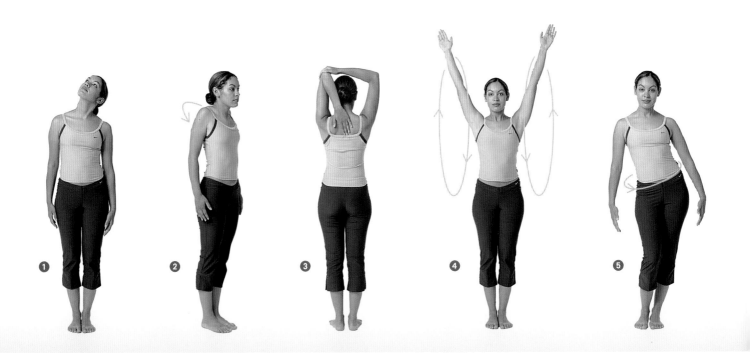

standing exercises

❶ neck stretch

Sit or stand comfortably with the back straight and arms and shoulders relaxed. Gently and slowly draw the head to the rear so that the chin is pointing upward. Hold 5–10 seconds. Then gently tilt to the right, again holding for 5–10 seconds. Repeat once more tilting to the left. The neck is a delicate area of the body, so slow and gentle movements are needed.

❶ **caution:** Avoid this exercise if prone to neck stiffness and aches.

✔ **benefits:** • Firms, tones, and relaxes the neck muscles • Increases the flexibility of the cervical vertebrae

❷ shoulder rolls

Stand with feet close together. Roll the shoulders around clockwise and then counterclockwise, three times each. Then, inhale deeply and on the exhalation relax the shoulders.

✔ **benefits:** • Tones the shoulder and upper back muscles

❸ upper arm stretch

Standing, raise both arms above the head with the palms facing forward. Fold the left arm to the rear, with the palm on the left scapula. Bend the right arm and with the right palm, cup the left elbow. Press down on the left elbow, drawing the left hand further down the back. Repeat with the other arm.

✔ **benefits:** • Tones the upper arms • Strengthens the wrists

❹ windmill

Stand with the feet close together and raise the right arm up straight. Propel the right arm down and up again. Continue so that the arm is rotating like a windmill. Rotate clockwise and then counterclockwise, doing five rotations in each direction. Repeat with the left arm. Then perform with both arms being propelled around clockwise and then counterclockwise. Breathe normally.

✔ **benefits:** • Tones the muscles in the upper back, chest, and arms • Limbers up the shoulder joints • Increases circulation to the fingers

There are many variations to the asanas (pages 38–123), some of which are shown in this book. This allows individuals of differing abilities to enjoy and explore the posture. When the main posture is difficult or uncomfortable to achieve, then a beginner-level variation can be practiced to develop the flexibility needed to attain the main posture. When the main posture is easily achieved, then the intermediate or advanced variation can be practiced.

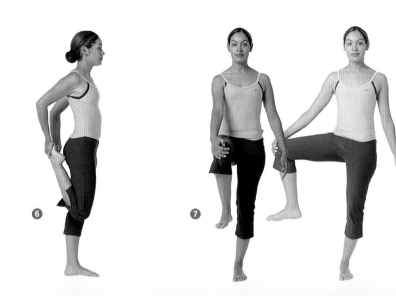
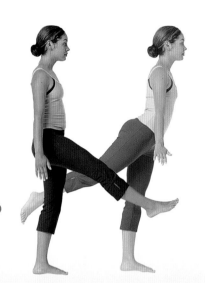

❺ hip rotation

Stand with feet close together and arms relaxed by the side. Keeping the back straight and feet in one spot, circle the hips around in a clockwise and then a counterclockwise direction, ten times.

benefits: • Limbers up the waist and hips

❻ thigh stretch

From a standing position, shift the weight onto the left foot and bend the right leg back. With one or both hands, press the right heel into the right buttock. Keep the thigh perpendicular. Hold for 5–10 seconds and return to standing. Repeat on the other side.

benefits: • Increases flexibility of the knee • Tones the legs • Stretches the sciatic nerve

❼ front-to-side leg raise

Stand with the feet close together and raise the right leg, with the knee flexed. Use one or both hands to press the knee up to the chest. Then reduce the bend at the knee and rotate the leg 90 degrees to the right. Hold for 5 seconds. Return to standing and repeat on the other side.

benefits: • Limbers up the pelvis • Tones the legs • Improves balance

❽ leg pendulum

Stand with the feet slightly apart and place your hands by your sides. Shift the weight onto the left leg and raise the right leg off the floor. In a smooth action, swing the leg to and fro. The sole of the foot should clear the floor as it swings past the left leg. Repeat on the other side.

benefits: • Limbers up the hips • Improves circulation to the toes • Tones the leg muscles • Improves balance

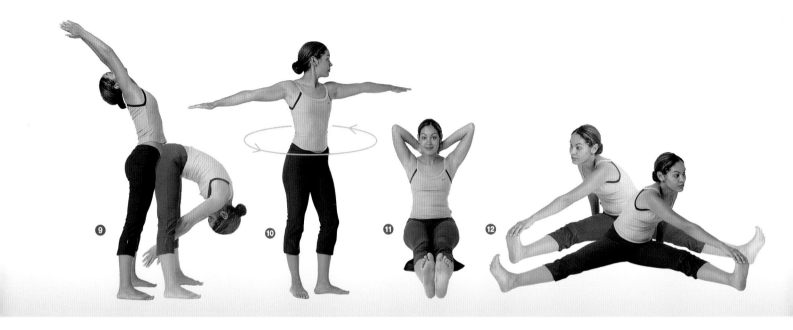

sitting exercises

❾ woodcutter

Stand with the feet shoulder-length apart. Inhale and raise the arms up, with palms pressed together. Arch the spine and bend the arms and trunk backward. Exhaling, swing the arms down through the legs, pressing the head in the same direction. Wait until the exhalation is complete and then inhale to repeat the upward swinging action. Continue for 30 seconds.

✔ **benefits:** • Increases spinal flexibility • Promotes deeper breathing

❿ spinning

Stand with the feet close together, and raise the arms up to shoulder level. Take a deep breath in and, on the exhalation, spin the entire body around in a clockwise direction. The feet revolve around in small shuffling steps to achieve the spinning action. Spin quickly seven times. Afterward, the room appears to move around. Wait for this to completely stop before spinning in the counterclockwise direction.

❶ **caution:** If you have high blood pressure or are prone to dizziness, you should not carry out this stretch.

✔ **benefits:** • Limbers up the legs, hips, and abdomen • Integrates and calms the nervous system

⓫ sitting arm and neck stretch

Sit either with the legs stretched out straight or cross-legged, and back erect. Interlock the fingers and straighten the arms out in front of the chest with the palms turned away from the body. Inhale and raise the linked arms up above the head. Bend at the elbow and bring the linked hands to rest behind the neck. Pull the elbows wide apart. Exhale, still cupping the neck, and bring the elbows forward to touch. Hold for 5–10 seconds and inhale to release. Repeat two more times. Then straighten the arms up again, and exhale to lower the arms and unlink the hands.

✔ **benefits:** • Reduces tension in the neck • Strengthens the arms and back

⓬ alternate hand-to-toe swing

Sit with the legs stretched forward and the back straight. Take the feet wide apart. Inhale and take the right hand to the left foot or ankle. Hold for 1–2 seconds, and exhale to release. Then take the left hand to the right foot. Repeat five more times.

✔ **benefits:** • Tones the back, legs, and abdomen

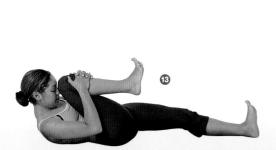

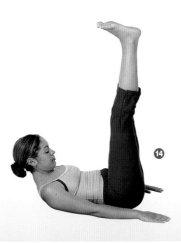

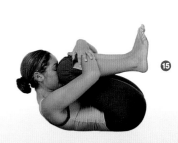

supine exercises

⑬ knee-to-head in supine

Lie on your back. Exhale and bend the right knee toward the chest. Clasp both arms around the knees and lift the head up toward the chest. Hold for 5–10 seconds, and release. Do the same, drawing the left knee to the forehead. Repeat this two more times.

✅ benefits: • Increases the blood circulation • Limbers up the hips • Tones the abdomen and legs

⑭ double leg raises

Lie stretched out on the floor with the arms by the side. Inhale, and slowly raise both legs by 90 degrees to a perpendicular position. Keep the legs straight. Exhale and slowly lower them back onto the floor. The head can also be raised by 60 degrees. If lifting both legs is uncomfortable, then raise one leg at a time.

❗ caution: If raising the head causes the shoulders to lift, then work only with the legs.

✅ benefits: • Limbers up the hips • Tones the leg muscles

⑮ rocking the body

Lie on the back and bend the knees toward the chest. Clasp arms around the knees and lift the head up toward the chest. Rock the body to and fro seven times, and then from side to side seven times. This relatively simple exercise has a beneficial effect on the nervous system. The rocking action compresses and invigorates the muscles and nerve endings, increasing awareness of the muscles.

✅ benefits: • Increases the blood circulation • Calms and focuses the mind

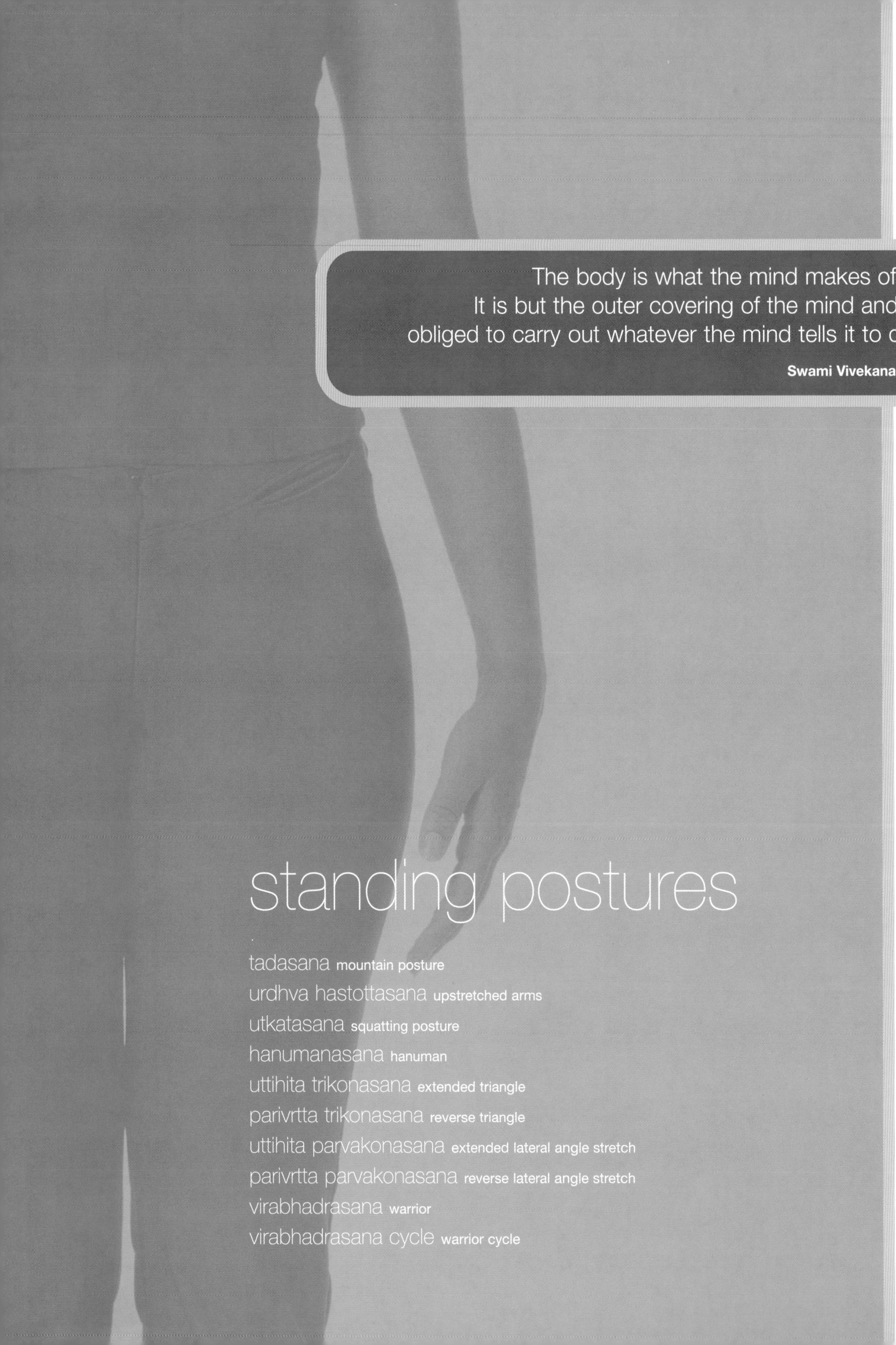

The body is what the mind makes of it.
It is but the outer covering of the mind and is
obliged to carry out whatever the mind tells it to do.

Swami Vivekananda

standing postures

tadasana mountain posture

urdhva hastottasana upstretched arms

utkatasana squatting posture

hanumanasana hanuman

uttihita trikonasana extended triangle

parivrtta trikonasana reverse triangle

uttihita parvakonasana extended lateral angle stretch

parivrtta parvakonasana reverse lateral angle stretch

virabhadrasana warrior

virabhadrasana cycle warrior cycle

tadasana mountain posture

Tada means "mountain." In Tadasana the body is erect like a mountain and the feet are planted firmly on the floor. The stance is poised rather than rigid. There will be a feeling of lightness in the body, as less effort is needed to maintain the position against gravity.

level: Beginner

benefits • Develops awareness of posture • Promotes spinal alignment • Improves general muscle tone

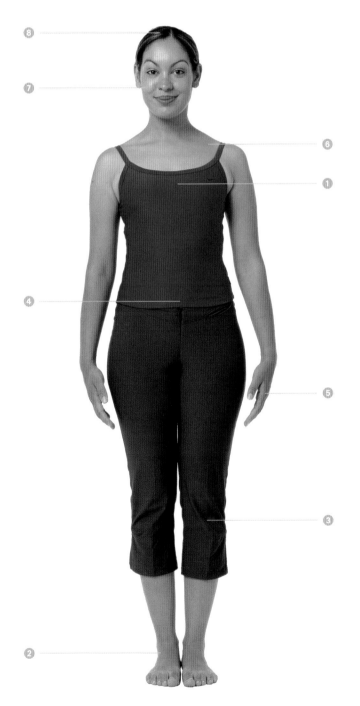

Tadasana is the starting (and ending) position of all standing postures. It is the body's natural standing position, allowing a steady and even flow of breath and enabling the mind to be focused.

❶ Begin by focusing on the breath. Steadily deepen the breath.

❷ Bring the feet close together so that the toes and heels are gently touching. Lift the toes up, spread them apart, and press them down. Press the heels likewise. Center the body so that the weight is evenly spread through the two feet.

❸ Tighten the knees by pulling up the kneecaps, stretching the back of the legs.

❹ Draw the stomach in and open the chest. Do not hollow out the back.

❺ Place the arms by the side of the body with the fingers pointing down.

❻ Exhaling, release the tension in the shoulders, lowering them.

❼ Relax the muscles of the face and throat.

❽ Imagine a string attached to the crown of the head, slowly pulling the body up.

urdhva hastottasana **upstretched arms posture**

Urdhva means "upward" and *hasta* means "hand." In urdhva hastottasana, the body is bent sideways, enabling the arms, spine, and legs to be lengthened and gently stretched.

level: Beginner

benefits • Improves posture and balance • Strengthens the wrist and ankles

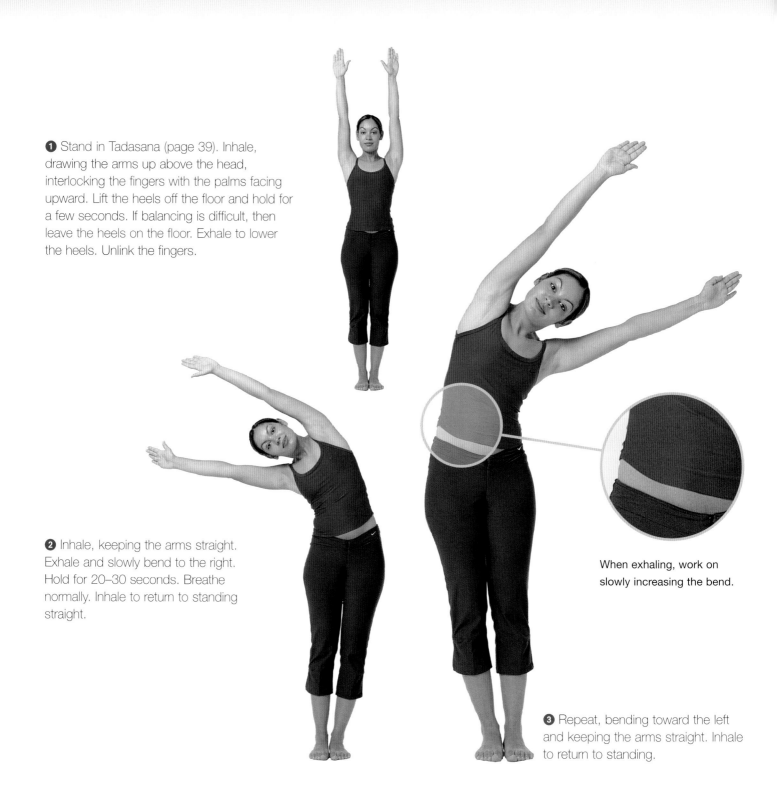

❶ Stand in Tadasana (page 39). Inhale, drawing the arms up above the head, interlocking the fingers with the palms facing upward. Lift the heels off the floor and hold for a few seconds. If balancing is difficult, then leave the heels on the floor. Exhale to lower the heels. Unlink the fingers.

❷ Inhale, keeping the arms straight. Exhale and slowly bend to the right. Hold for 20–30 seconds. Breathe normally. Inhale to return to standing straight.

When exhaling, work on slowly increasing the bend.

❸ Repeat, bending toward the left and keeping the arms straight. Inhale to return to standing.

utkatasana squatting posture

Utkata means "powerful" or "mighty." Gheranda Samhita lists Utkatasana as one of the thirty-two important Hatha yoga asanas. In the Indian subcontinent, this position is often used for sitting. The variation of squatting on tiptoes is used for some of the Tantric breathing exercises to control sexual energies.

level: Beginner

benefits • Strengthens the legs and ankles • Tones the abdominal muscles • Relieves constipation

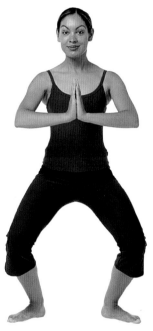

❷ Now press the elbows against the knees to keep them apart. Draw the head upward and straighten the back. Hold for 20 seconds. Inhale to return to standing erect.

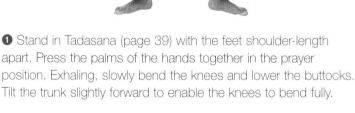

❶ Stand in Tadasana (page 39) with the feet shoulder-length apart. Press the palms of the hands together in the prayer position. Exhaling, slowly bend the knees and lower the buttocks. Tilt the trunk slightly forward to enable the knees to bend fully.

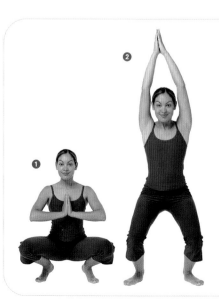

VARIATIONS

❶ **beginner:** The feet are about shoulder-length apart. Lift the heels off the floor and bend the knees, weight-bearing on the toes and sitting on the heels. The palms are pressed together at chest level.

❷ **intermediate:** This variation is known as Sahaj utkatasana or "chair posture," as it resembles sitting on an invisible chair. The feet are close together. The arms are stretched above the head with palms pressed together. Bend the knees and lower the body.

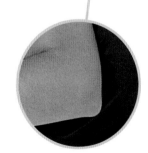

Press the elbow against the legs to stretch the legs farther apart.

hanumanasana **hanuman posture**

Hanuman is a Hindu deity renowned for his wisdom and strength. Traditionally, the Hanumanasana involves performing a side leg split. However, as this is difficult to achieve at first, the posture has been adapted here.

level: Beginner

caution: Perform the posture on a blanket if this hurts the knees.

benefits • Tones the legs and arms • Improves circulation to the feet • Increases flexibility at the hips

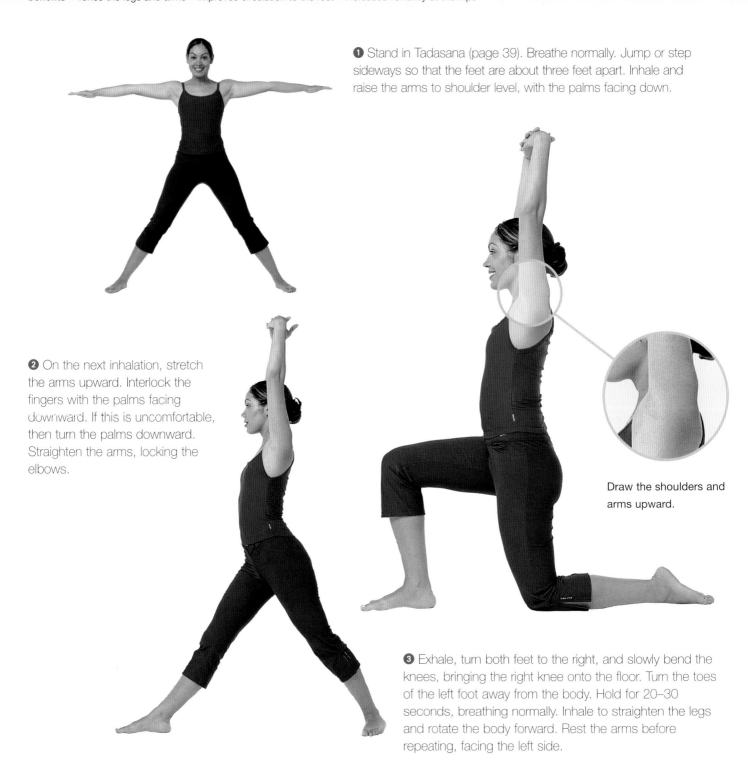

❶ Stand in Tadasana (page 39). Breathe normally. Jump or step sideways so that the feet are about three feet apart. Inhale and raise the arms to shoulder level, with the palms facing down.

❷ On the next inhalation, stretch the arms upward. Interlock the fingers with the palms facing downward. If this is uncomfortable, then turn the palms downward. Straighten the arms, locking the elbows.

Draw the shoulders and arms upward.

❸ Exhale, turn both feet to the right, and slowly bend the knees, bringing the right knee onto the floor. Turn the toes of the left foot away from the body. Hold for 20–30 seconds, breathing normally. Inhale to straighten the legs and rotate the body forward. Rest the arms before repeating, facing the left side.

uttihita trikonasana **extended triangle**

Uttihita means "extended" or "stretched" and *trikona* means "triangle." Uttihita trikonasana is a posture intended to stretch the side of the body. The hips should face squarely forward. Don't be tempted to bend the hips and trunk forward to place the hand on the floor.

level: Beginner

caution: If rotating the neck to look up is uncomfortable or painful, look forward instead.

benefits • Regulates the digestive system • Strengthens the ankles and legs

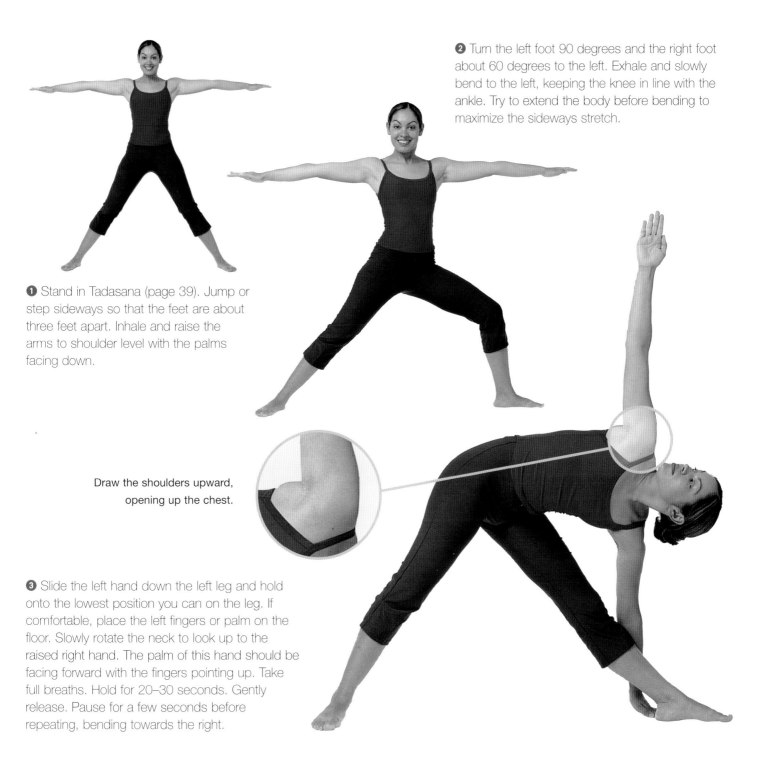

❷ Turn the left foot 90 degrees and the right foot about 60 degrees to the left. Exhale and slowly bend to the left, keeping the knee in line with the ankle. Try to extend the body before bending to maximize the sideways stretch.

❶ Stand in Tadasana (page 39). Jump or step sideways so that the feet are about three feet apart. Inhale and raise the arms to shoulder level with the palms facing down.

Draw the shoulders upward, opening up the chest.

❸ Slide the left hand down the left leg and hold onto the lowest position you can on the leg. If comfortable, place the left fingers or palm on the floor. Slowly rotate the neck to look up to the raised right hand. The palm of this hand should be facing forward with the fingers pointing up. Take full breaths. Hold for 20–30 seconds. Gently release. Pause for a few seconds before repeating, bending towards the right.

parivrtta trikonasana reverse triangle posture

Parivrtta means "reverse" or "rotated" and *trikona* means "triangle." Parivrtta trikonasana is the counterposture to Uttihita trikonasana (page 43), giving an extensive stretch to the hamstring and calf muscles. If balancing is difficult, then practice the posture against a wall.

level: Beginner/Intermediate

caution: The organs of the abdomen are strongly compressed. Do not hold if there is any discomfort at the abdomen.

benefits • Regulates the digestive system • Massages the internal organs, such as the liver

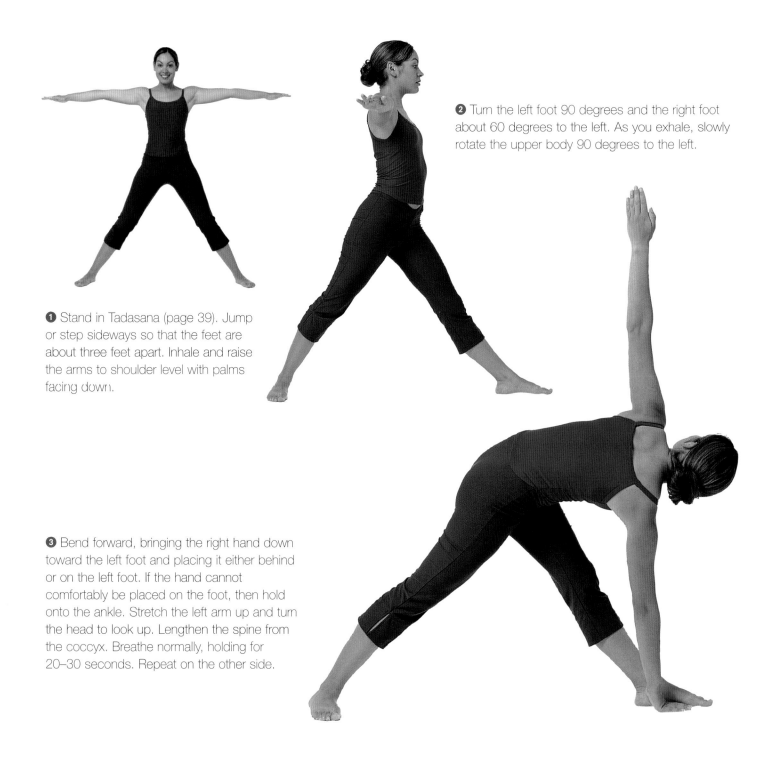

❷ Turn the left foot 90 degrees and the right foot about 60 degrees to the left. As you exhale, slowly rotate the upper body 90 degrees to the left.

❶ Stand in Tadasana (page 39). Jump or step sideways so that the feet are about three feet apart. Inhale and raise the arms to shoulder level with palms facing down.

❸ Bend forward, bringing the right hand down toward the left foot and placing it either behind or on the left foot. If the hand cannot comfortably be placed on the foot, then hold onto the ankle. Stretch the left arm up and turn the head to look up. Lengthen the spine from the coccyx. Breathe normally, holding for 20–30 seconds. Repeat on the other side.

uttihita parvsakonasana **extended lateral angle stretch**

Parvsa means "side" or "flank" and *kona* is "an angle." This standing posture strongly stretches the side of the body. If balancing is difficult, practice the posture against a wall. As in the Triangle posture, the hips face squarely forward.

level: Intermediate

caution: The side of the abdomen is compressed. Do not hold if there is any discomfort at the abdomen.

benefits • Regulates the digestive system • Strengthens the ankles and legs

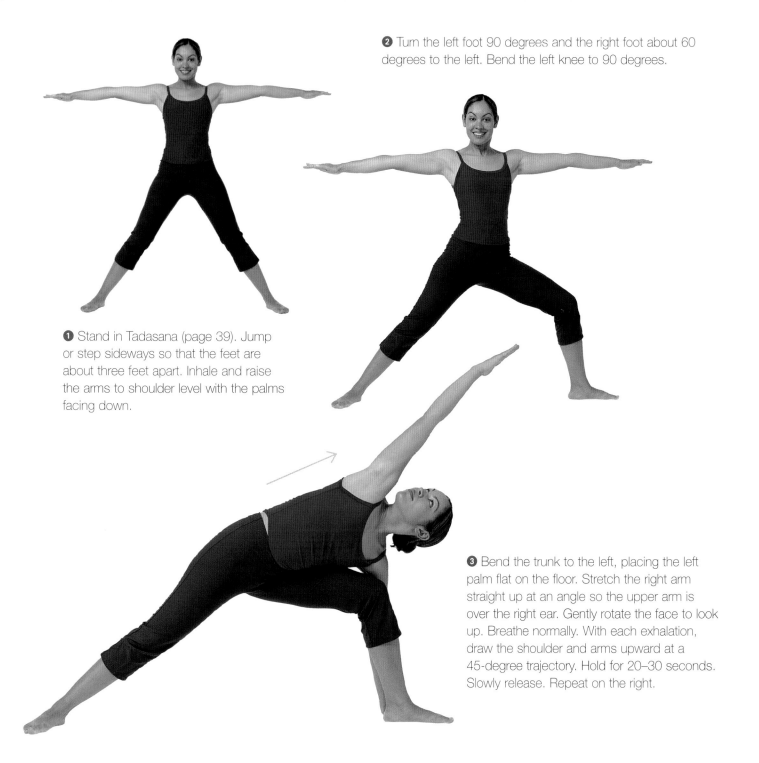

❷ Turn the left foot 90 degrees and the right foot about 60 degrees to the left. Bend the left knee to 90 degrees.

❶ Stand in Tadasana (page 39). Jump or step sideways so that the feet are about three feet apart. Inhale and raise the arms to shoulder level with the palms facing down.

❸ Bend the trunk to the left, placing the left palm flat on the floor. Stretch the right arm straight up at an angle so the upper arm is over the right ear. Gently rotate the face to look up. Breathe normally. With each exhalation, draw the shoulder and arms upward at a 45-degree trajectory. Hold for 20–30 seconds. Slowly release. Repeat on the right.

parivrtta parvakonasana reverse lateral angle stretch

Parivrtta means "rotated" or "reverse" and *parsvakona* means "lateral angle." Parivrtta parvakonasana requires considerable suppleness, as the trunk is rotated 180 degrees from its starting position. If balancing is difficult, practice the posture against the wall.

level: Intermediate/Advanced

caution: The compression in the abdomen is intense. Do not hold if there is any discomfort at the abdomen.

benefits • Regulates the digestive system • Relieves constipation • Strengthens the ankles and legs

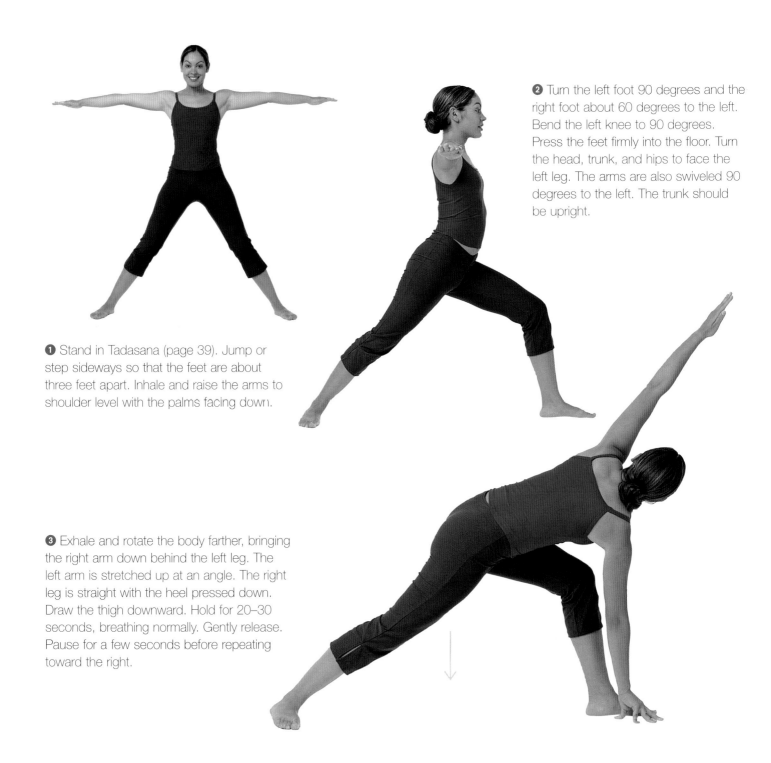

❶ Stand in Tadasana (page 39). Jump or step sideways so that the feet are about three feet apart. Inhale and raise the arms to shoulder level with the palms facing down.

❷ Turn the left foot 90 degrees and the right foot about 60 degrees to the left. Bend the left knee to 90 degrees. Press the feet firmly into the floor. Turn the head, trunk, and hips to face the left leg. The arms are also swiveled 90 degrees to the left. The trunk should be upright.

❸ Exhale and rotate the body farther, bringing the right arm down behind the left leg. The left arm is stretched up at an angle. The right leg is straight with the heel pressed down. Draw the thigh downward. Hold for 20–30 seconds, breathing normally. Gently release. Pause for a few seconds before repeating toward the right.

virabhadrasana **warrior posture**

Virabhadra is a legendary Indian warrior. To avenge the death of his beautiful wife Parvati, Lord Shiva manifested Virabhadra to fight his battle. Virabhadrasana is a powerful stretch that increases confidence, promotes self-esteem, and combats nervousness and fatigue.

level: Beginner/Intermediate

caution: Avoid this posture if prone to high blood pressure or heart problems.

benefits • Expands the chest • Strengthens the legs and back • Focuses the mind

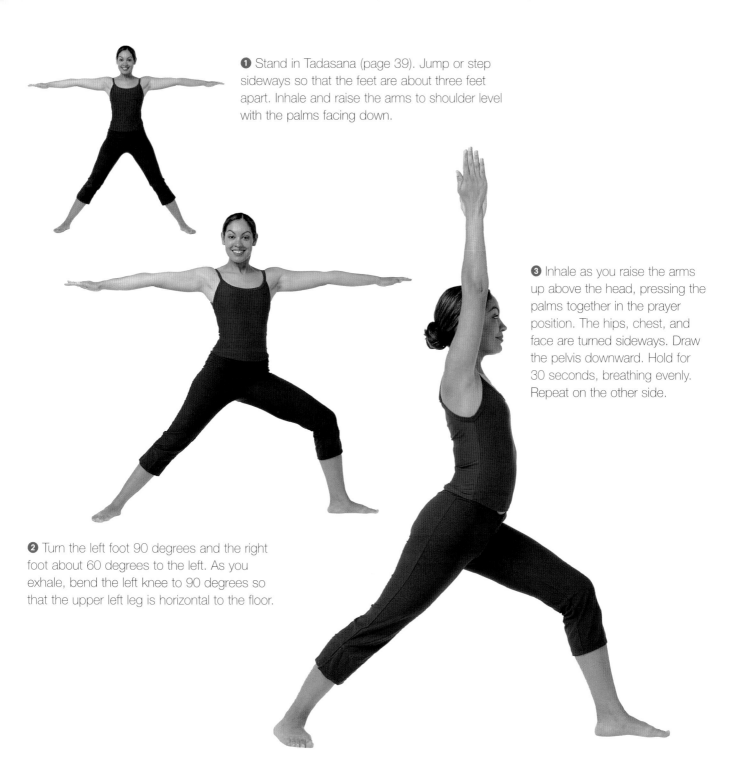

❶ Stand in Tadasana (page 39). Jump or step sideways so that the feet are about three feet apart. Inhale and raise the arms to shoulder level with the palms facing down.

❸ Inhale as you raise the arms up above the head, pressing the palms together in the prayer position. The hips, chest, and face are turned sideways. Draw the pelvis downward. Hold for 30 seconds, breathing evenly. Repeat on the other side.

❷ Turn the left foot 90 degrees and the right foot about 60 degrees to the left. As you exhale, bend the left knee to 90 degrees so that the upper left leg is horizontal to the floor.

virabhadrasana cycle **warrior cycle**

This cycle involves moving through four variations of Virabhadrasana. The lower part of the body is firmly grounded and held static, while the upper body moves slowly and purposefully through the different arm and trunk positions.

level: Beginner/Intermediate

caution: Avoid if you are prone to high blood pressure or back and neck problems.

benefits • Regulates the digestive system • Strengthens the ankles and legs • Develops confidence

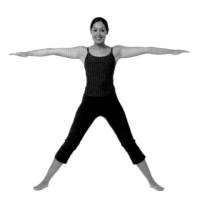

❶ Stand in Tadasana (page 39). Step sideways so that the feet are about three feet apart. Inhale and raise the arms sideways to shoulder level with the palms facing down.

viradbhadrasana 1

❷ Turn the left foot 90 degrees and the right foot 60 degrees to the left. Bend the left knee so that the thigh is parallel to the floor. Firm the legs and press the feet firmly into the floor. The position of the legs is held firm for the next three Virabhadrasana variations. Hold for 10 seconds, breathing normally.

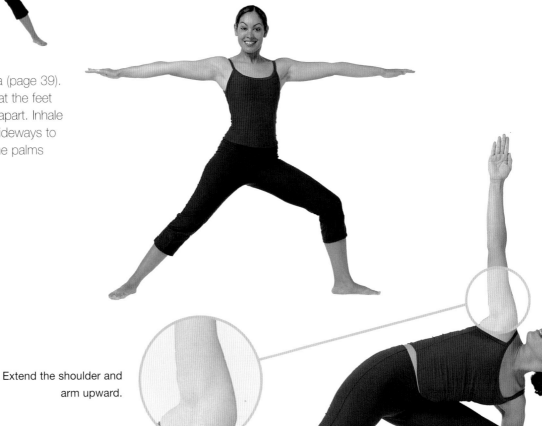

Extend the shoulder and arm upward.

viradbhadrasana 2

❸ Exhale and slowly rotate the trunk and arms 90 degrees to the right. Place the left hand on the floor and stretch the right arm up, palm facing forward. Look forward or up. Hold for 15 seconds, breathing normally.

viradbhadrasana 3

❹ Exhaling, bring the right palm down beside the left foot. Breathe in, then on the exhalation, raise the trunk to align vertically and bring both arms up to shoulder level. Either press the palms together or have them slightly apart. Hold for 10 seconds.

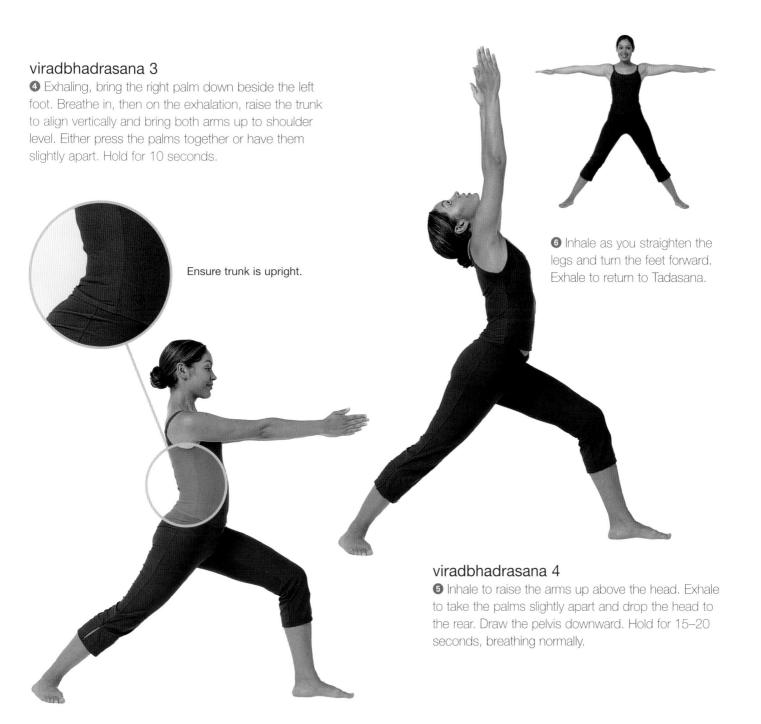

Ensure trunk is upright.

❻ Inhale as you straighten the legs and turn the feet forward. Exhale to return to Tadasana.

viradbhadrasana 4

❺ Inhale to raise the arms up above the head. Exhale to take the palms slightly apart and drop the head to the rear. Draw the pelvis downward. Hold for 15–20 seconds, breathing normally.

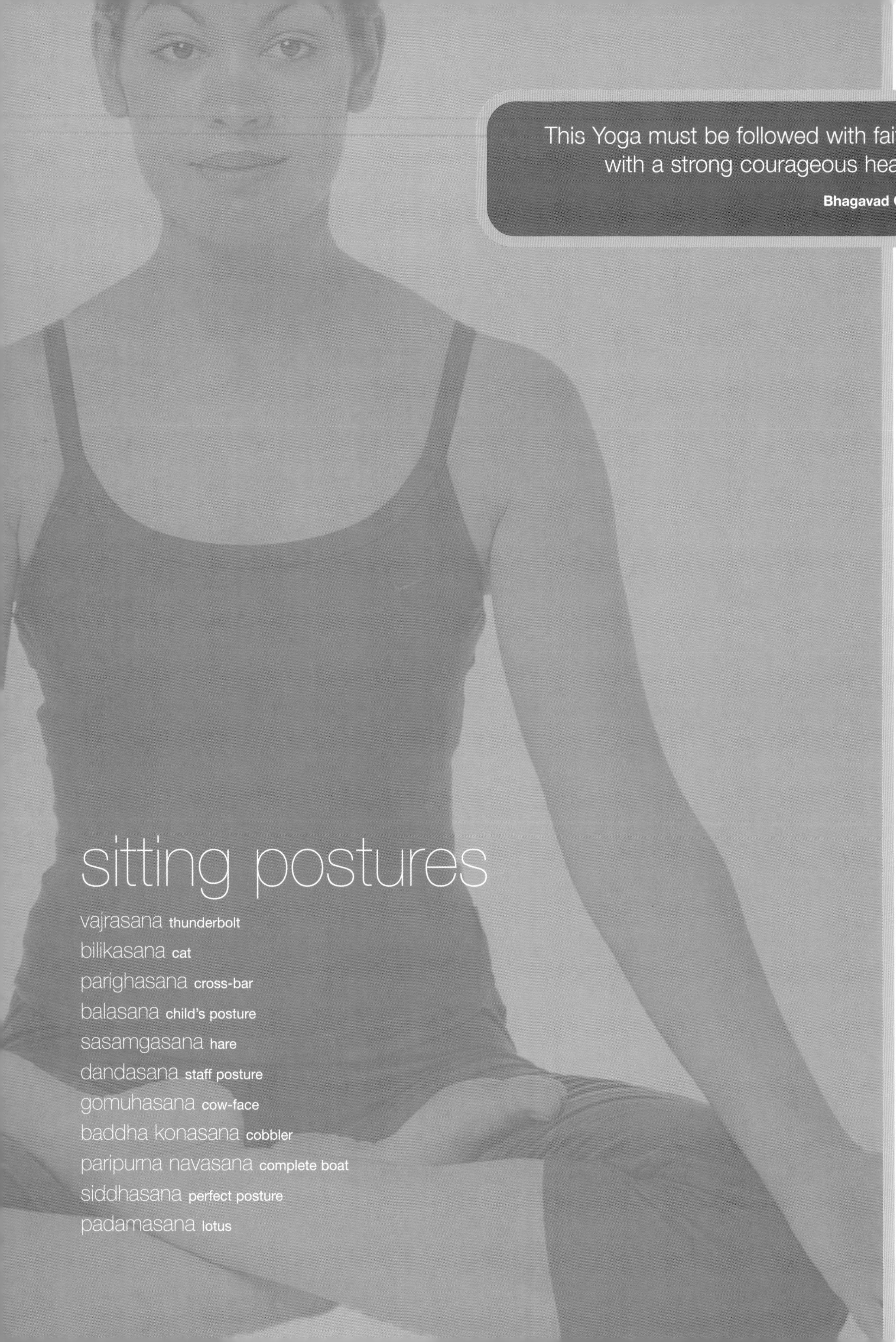

This Yoga must be followed with faith,
with a strong courageous heart.

Bhagavad Gita

sitting postures

vajrasana thunderbolt

bilikasana cat

parighasana cross-bar

balasana child's posture

sasamgasana hare

dandasana staff posture

gomuhasana cow-face

baddha konasana cobbler

paripurna navasana complete boat

siddhasana perfect posture

padamasana lotus

vajrasana thunderbolt posture

Vajra means "thunderbolt." The god of rain, Indra, used the thunderbolt as a weapon. Vajrasana is also called "Adamantine" or "Diamond." B. K. S. Iyengar calls this Virasana or "Hero posture." Vajrasana grounds the body like a rock, bringing calmness and serenity to the mind. It is a good starting position for many sitting postures.

level: Beginner

caution: Avoid the final position if uncomfortable and continue to sit on the heels. Practice this position to enable the knees and ankles to become supple.

benefits • Tones the thighs, knees, and ankles • Aids digestion when practiced after a meal • Calms the mind

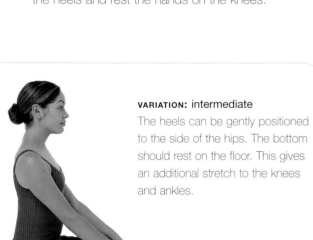

❶ Stand in Tadasana (page 39). Come to a kneeling position with the toes pointing away. Relax the shoulders and arms. Sit back on the heels and rest the hands on the knees.

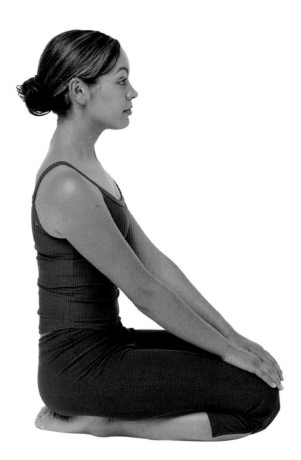

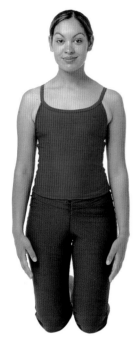

VARIATION: intermediate
The heels can be gently positioned to the side of the hips. The bottom should rest on the floor. This gives an additional stretch to the knees and ankles.

❸ Sit with the back erect, looking forward. Breathe evenly and deeply. Avoid hollowing the back. Hold for 30–60 seconds, breathing evenly.

bilikasana cat posture

Bilika means "cat" or "kitten." The graceful movements of the cat are mimicked in this posture. This is a relaxing stretch, which encourages deep breathing. Bilikasana is a good counterposture to Uttanasana (page 78). It is also a good stretch to precede prone postures such as Dhanurasana (page 74–75).

level: Beginner

caution: Practice on a blanket if weight-bearing on knees is painful.

benefits • Promotes flexibility of the spine • Strengthens the back and pelvic area

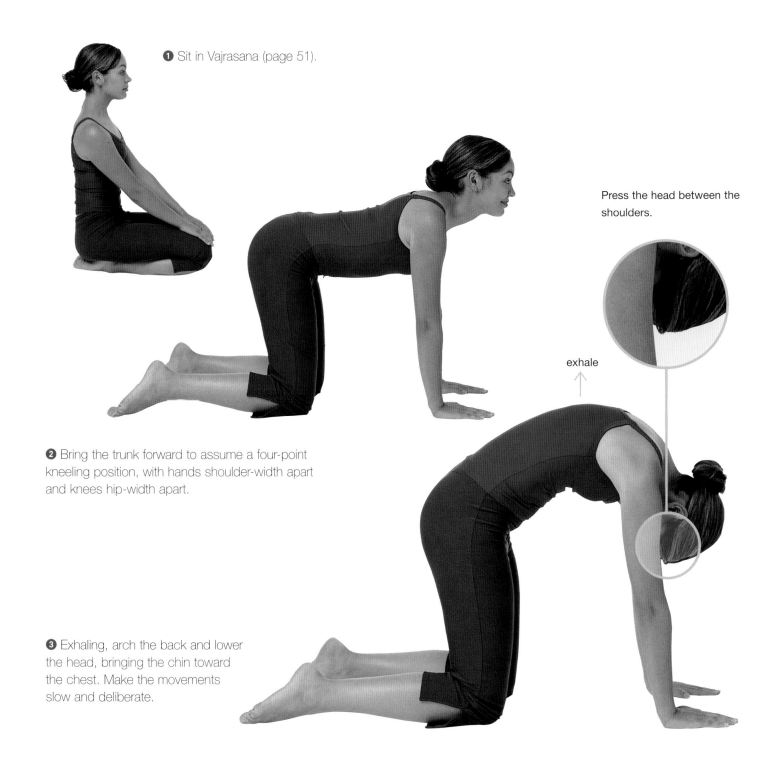

❶ Sit in Vajrasana (page 51).

Press the head between the shoulders.

exhale

❷ Bring the trunk forward to assume a four-point kneeling position, with hands shoulder-width apart and knees hip-width apart.

❸ Exhaling, arch the back and lower the head, bringing the chin toward the chest. Make the movements slow and deliberate.

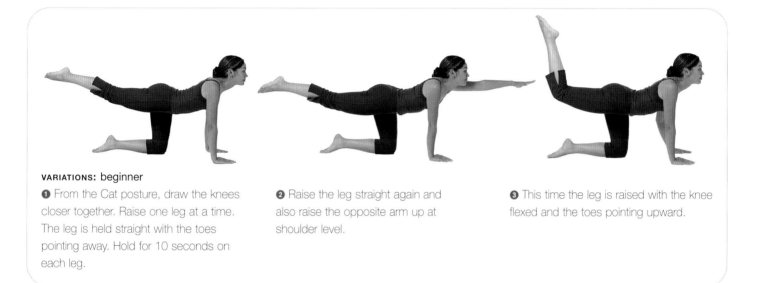

VARIATIONS: beginner

❶ From the Cat posture, draw the knees closer together. Raise one leg at a time. The leg is held straight with the toes pointing away. Hold for 10 seconds on each leg.

❷ Raise the leg straight again and also raise the opposite arm up at shoulder level.

❸ This time the leg is raised with the knee flexed and the toes pointing upward.

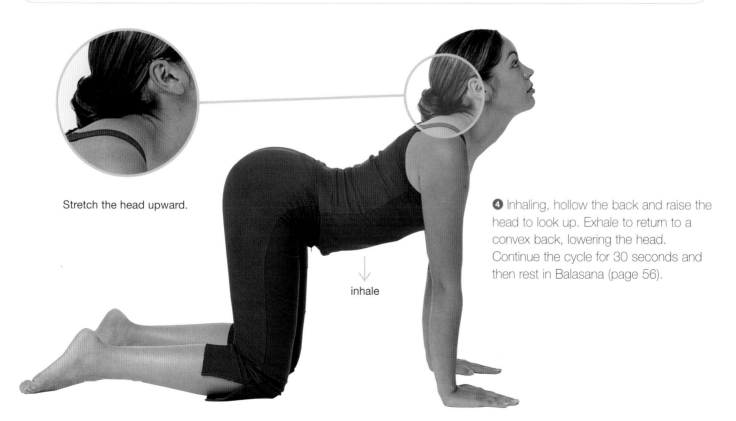

Stretch the head upward.

inhale

❹ Inhaling, hollow the back and raise the head to look up. Exhale to return to a convex back, lowering the head. Continue the cycle for 30 seconds and then rest in Balasana (page 56).

parighasana **cross-bar posture**

Parigha means "bar for securing a gate." Parighasana gives a powerful sideways stretch as the body is curved in an arc.

level: Beginner

caution: Practice on a blanket if the posture hurts the knees.

benefits • Limbers up the hips • Tones the abdomen and legs • Trims the waist • Massages the abdominal organs and spinal nerves

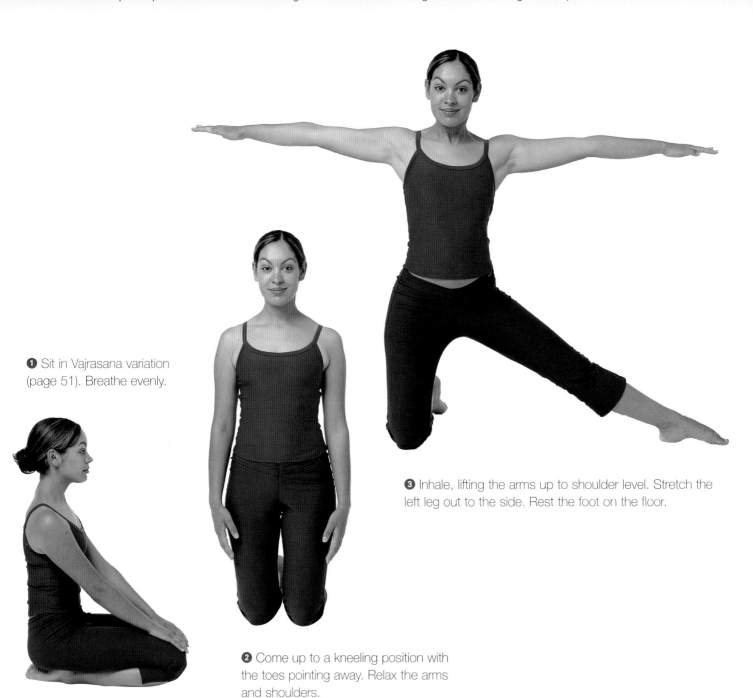

❶ Sit in Vajrasana variation (page 51). Breathe evenly.

❸ Inhale, lifting the arms up to shoulder level. Stretch the left leg out to the side. Rest the foot on the floor.

❷ Come up to a kneeling position with the toes pointing away. Relax the arms and shoulders.

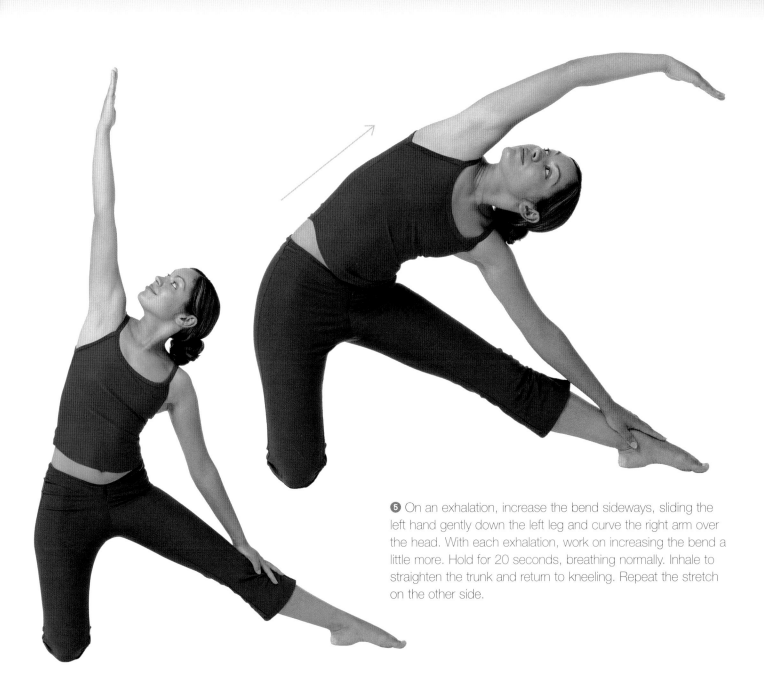

5 On an exhalation, increase the bend sideways, sliding the left hand gently down the left leg and curve the right arm over the head. With each exhalation, work on increasing the bend a little more. Hold for 20 seconds, breathing normally. Inhale to straighten the trunk and return to kneeling. Repeat the stretch on the other side.

4 Exhale, bending the trunk sideways, placing the left hand on the left knee and stretching the right arm up. Turn the head to look up at the hand stretching up. Hold for 10 seconds, breathing normally.

balasana child's posture

Bala means "child" or "infant." Balasana is a relaxation posture. In this position the spine is bent forward 110 degrees, providing an excellent counterstretch to those stretches involving a backward arch of the spine.

level: Beginner

benefits • Stretches the lumbar vertebrae • Relaxes the spinal ligaments • Relieves tired feet • Nourishes the facial skin and scalp • Reduces fatigue

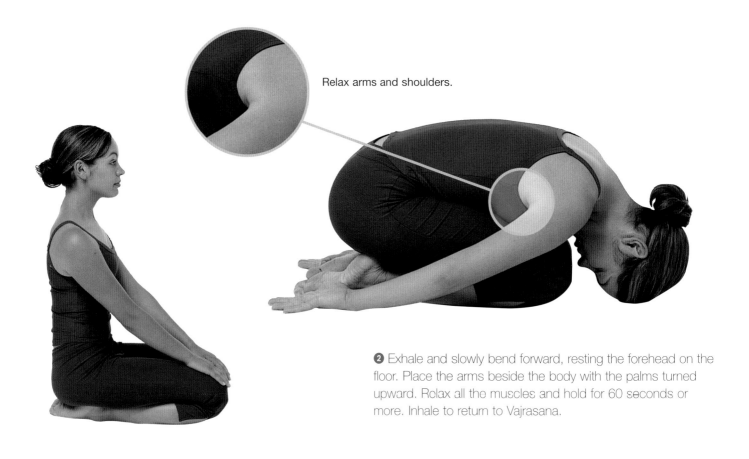

Relax arms and shoulders.

❷ Exhale and slowly bend forward, resting the forehead on the floor. Place the arms beside the body with the palms turned upward. Relax all the muscles and hold for 60 seconds or more. Inhale to return to Vajrasana.

❶ Sit in Vajrasana (page 51).

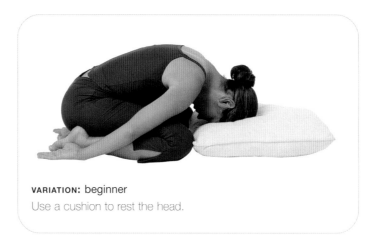

VARIATION: beginner
Use a cushion to rest the head.

sasamgasana **hare posture**

Sasa means "hare" or "moon" and *samga* means "closure" or "coming together." Sasamgasana is a useful posture to practice before inverted postures or meditation practice. The flow of blood to the face, neck, and brain is increased, enabling the mind to become calm and focused.

level: Beginner

caution: If you have high blood pressure or a heart problem, you should avoid this posture.

benefits • Relaxes the shoulders • Relieves mental fatigue and refreshes the brain • Benefits the sinuses

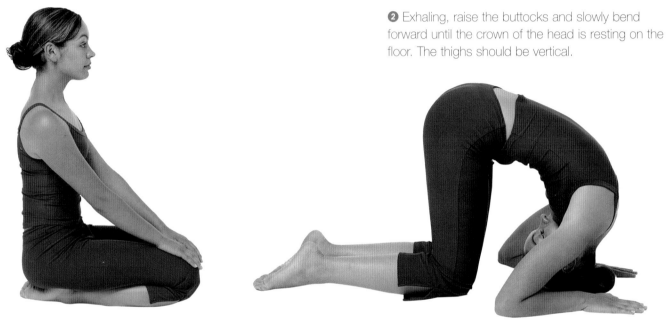

❷ Exhaling, raise the buttocks and slowly bend forward until the crown of the head is resting on the floor. The thighs should be vertical.

❶ Sit in Vajrasana (page 51). Relax the shoulders and rest the hands on the thighs.

Pull hips forward to ensure thighs are perpendicular to the floor.

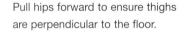

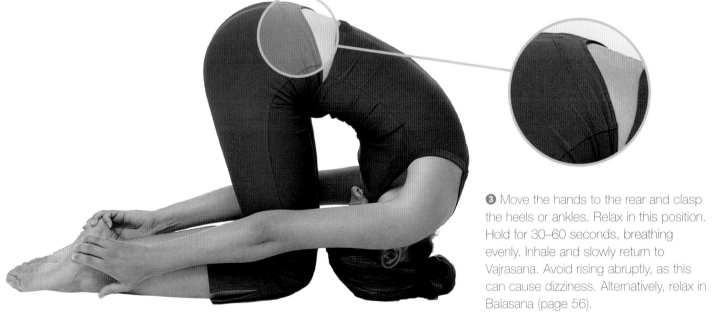

❸ Move the hands to the rear and clasp the heels or ankles. Relax in this position. Hold for 30–60 seconds, breathing evenly. Inhale and slowly return to Vajrasana. Avoid rising abruptly, as this can cause dizziness. Alternatively, relax in Balasana (page 56).

dandasana staff posture

Danda means "staff" or "rod." In Dandasana, the back is straight and erect. It is the starting position of many sitting postures. The practice of this posture develops a good pattern of sitting on a chair or sofa.

level: Beginner

caution: If you have a tendency to curve the back, then sit on a folded blanket or against a wall for additional support.

benefits • Increases awareness of posture • Tones the legs

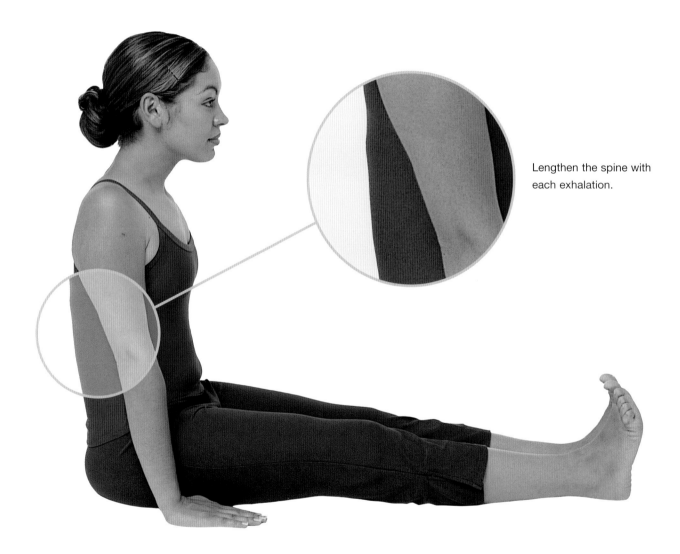

Lengthen the spine with each exhalation.

❶ Sit on the floor or mat with the legs stretched out straight in front. Press the knees down and point the toes up. Press the palms on the floor beside the hips. Lengthen the spine and work on sitting upright. Center the head and look forward. Breathe normally, holding for 20–30 seconds.

gomukhasana **cow-face posture**

Go means "cow" and *mukha* means "face." In Gomukhasana the energy channels of ha and tha are crossed, promoting equilibrium in the body. The posture is based on the cow's face, as the feet resemble the shape of the cow's horns.

level: Beginner/Intermediate

practice: If you find sitting with legs crossed difficult, sit in Vajrasana (page 51). If linking the fingers is difficult, clasp a towel or scarf between both hands.

benefits • Tones the upper arms and shoulders • Cleanses the lungs • Calms the mind

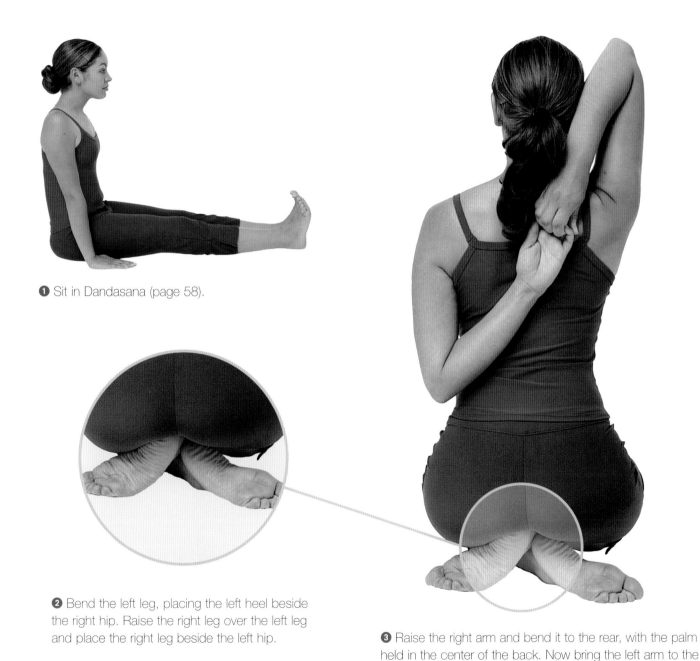

❶ Sit in Dandasana (page 58).

❷ Bend the left leg, placing the left heel beside the right hip. Raise the right leg over the left leg and place the right leg beside the left hip.

❸ Raise the right arm and bend it to the rear, with the palm held in the center of the back. Now bring the left arm to the rear from the waist. Clasp the fingers together and stretch the elbows in opposite directions. Sit erect with the head centered, looking ahead. Hold for 10–20 seconds, breathing deeply. Release slowly. Repeat with the opposite limbs.

baddha konasana **cobbler posture**

Baddha means "caught" or "restrained"; *kona* means "angle." In Baddha konasana, the legs are angled inward with the soles of the feet pressed together. It is the traditional position that the Indian cobbler assumes when working. The posture keeps the kidneys, prostate, and urinary bladder healthy.

level: Beginner

benefits • Tones the legs and pelvic muscles • Regulates the function of the kidney, ovaries, and prostate glands • Increases flexibility at the hips and ankles

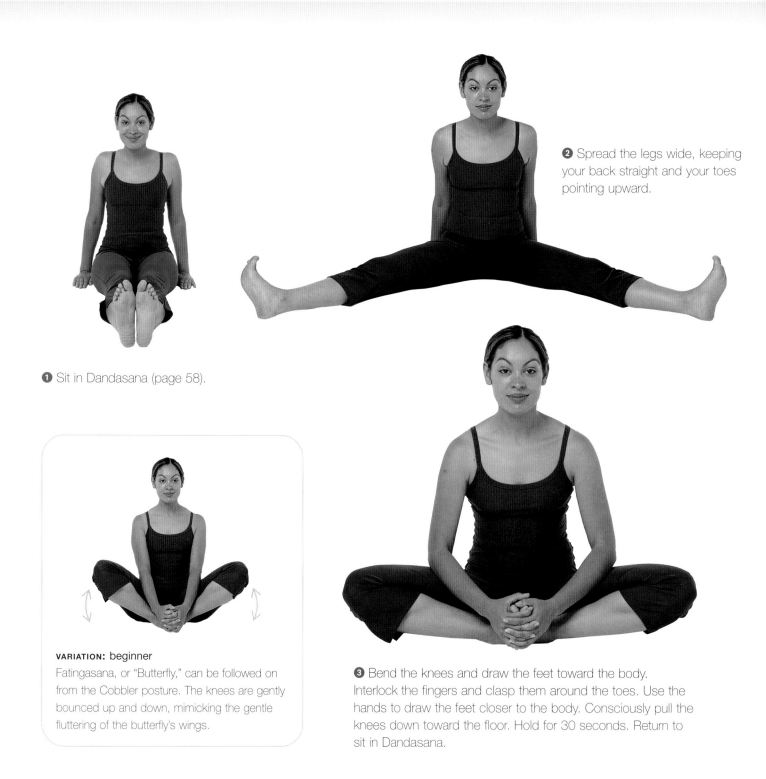

❷ Spread the legs wide, keeping your back straight and your toes pointing upward.

❶ Sit in Dandasana (page 58).

VARIATION: beginner

Fatingasana, or "Butterfly," can be followed on from the Cobbler posture. The knees are gently bounced up and down, mimicking the gentle fluttering of the butterfly's wings.

❸ Bend the knees and draw the feet toward the body. Interlock the fingers and clasp them around the toes. Use the hands to draw the feet closer to the body. Consciously pull the knees down toward the floor. Hold for 30 seconds. Return to sit in Dandasana.

paripurna navasana **complete boat posture**

Paripurna means "complete" and *nava* means "boat." Paripurna navasana resembles a boat with oars. The back and the stomach muscles are activated to hold this posture. Strengthening these muscles is particularly beneficial for preventing lower back problems.

level: Beginner/Intermediate

caution: If prone to lower back pain, avoid this posture. If the posture is difficult because of weak stomach muscles, then practice the variation.

benefits • Strengthens the stomach and back muscles • Revitalizes the spine

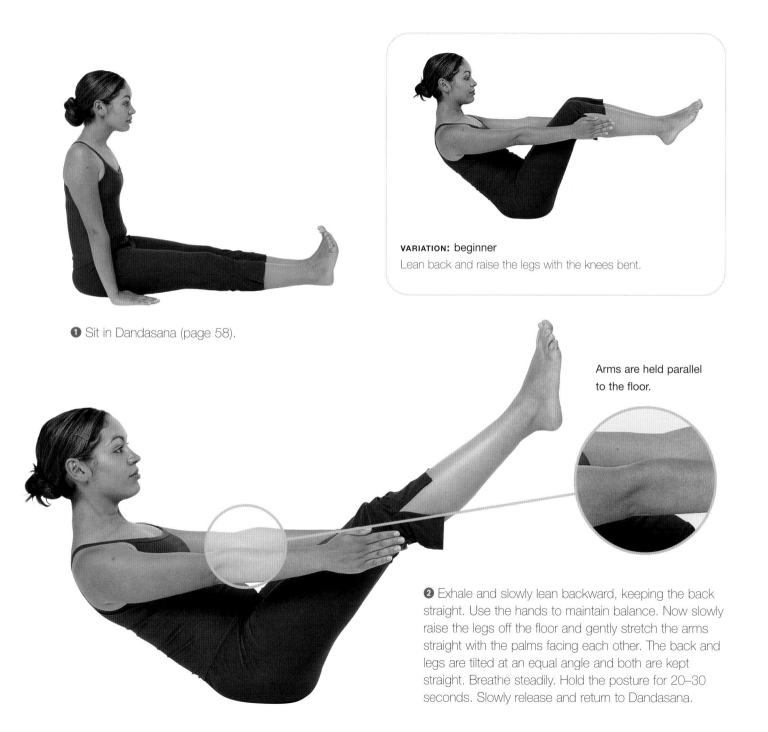

VARIATION: beginner
Lean back and raise the legs with the knees bent.

❶ Sit in Dandasana (page 58).

Arms are held parallel to the floor.

❷ Exhale and slowly lean backward, keeping the back straight. Use the hands to maintain balance. Now slowly raise the legs off the floor and gently stretch the arms straight with the palms facing each other. The back and legs are tilted at an equal angle and both are kept straight. Breathe steadily. Hold the posture for 20–30 seconds. Slowly release and return to Dandasana.

siddhasana **perfect posture**

Siddha means "proficient" or "perfect." Siddhas are yogis or sages who possess supernatural faculties. Siddhasana is recommended for the practice of pranayama and meditation.

level: Beginner

caution: If the positioning of the feet is uncomfortable, practice sitting in Sukhasana (cross-legged).

benefits • Increases pelvic mobility • Strengthens the ankle, knee, and hip joints • Calms the nervous system • Relaxes the mind and body

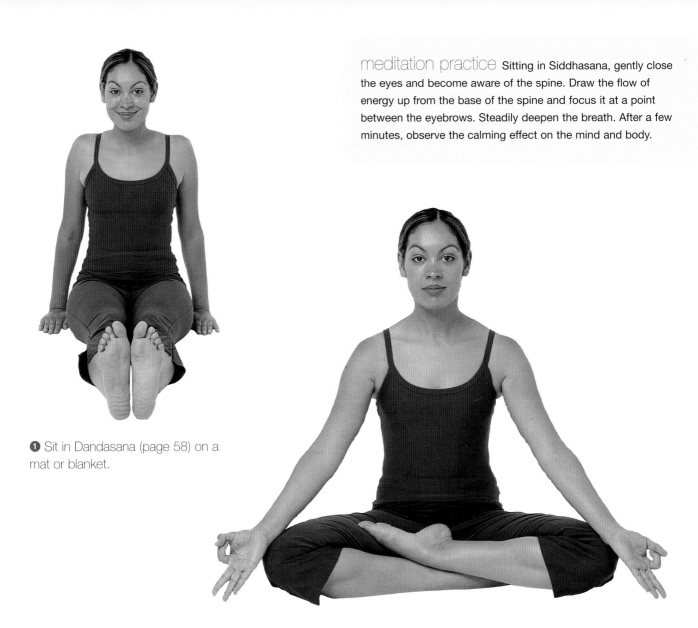

meditation practice Sitting in Siddhasana, gently close the eyes and become aware of the spine. Draw the flow of energy up from the base of the spine and focus it at a point between the eyebrows. Steadily deepen the breath. After a few minutes, observe the calming effect on the mind and body.

❶ Sit in Dandasana (page 58) on a mat or blanket.

❷ Draw the right foot toward the body and place the heel against the perineum (the area just below the reproductive organs). The left leg is then folded and the heel pulled against the pubic bone above the reproductive organs. The sole of the left foot is turned upward and the toes tucked into the fold of the right leg. The left heel should be resting above the left thigh.

padmasana **lotus posture**

Padma means "lotus." Padmasana is the classical posture used for the practice of pranayama and meditation. For many people this posture is one of the most difficult to master. Once mastered, Padmasana is one of the most relaxing postures. The lower body is compact, giving stability to the upper body. The back is erect and the mind is able to remain alert.

level: Beginner

caution: Never force the feet into this posture. First become accustomed to sitting cross-legged. Initially begin with Ardha padmasana, or "Half-lotus" posture.

benefits: Increases pelvic mobility • Massages the abdominal organs • Increases circulation in the lumbar region • Strengthens ankle, knee, and hip joints

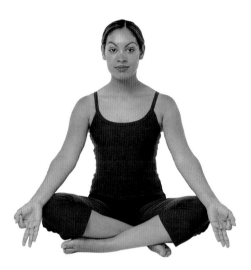

❶ Begin by sitting cross-legged on a blanket or mat. Exhale, bending the right knee and placing the right foot on the left thigh with the sole of the foot turned upward. Use the hands to draw the foot up against the groin.

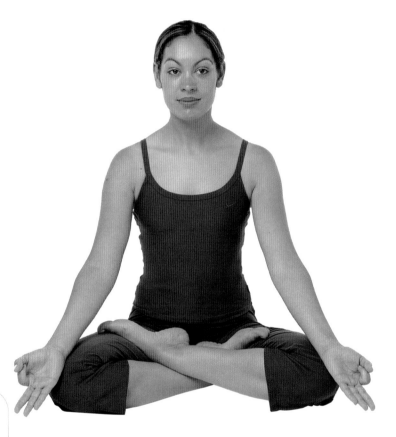

❷ Bend the left knee and place the left foot on top of the right thigh with the sole of the foot turned upward. Again use the hands to draw the foot up against the groin. Bring the knees closer together. Sit with the back straight. Either rest the hands on the thighs or stretch them out straight on the knee. The palm is facing up and the thumb and index finger are linked up in the jnana mudra (page 33). Hold for 30–60 seconds. To emerge from the posture, use the hands to lift the feet off the thighs. Rotate the ankles to release tension. Alternate the position of the feet the next time you practice.

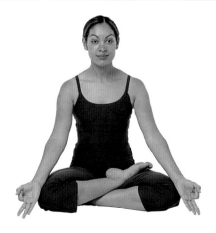

VARIATION: beginner

In Ardha padmasana (half lotus), one foot is raised onto the opposite thigh, while the other foot is tucked under the thigh. The soles of both feet are turned upward.

Yoga is the producer of the greatest happiness.

Bhagavad Gita

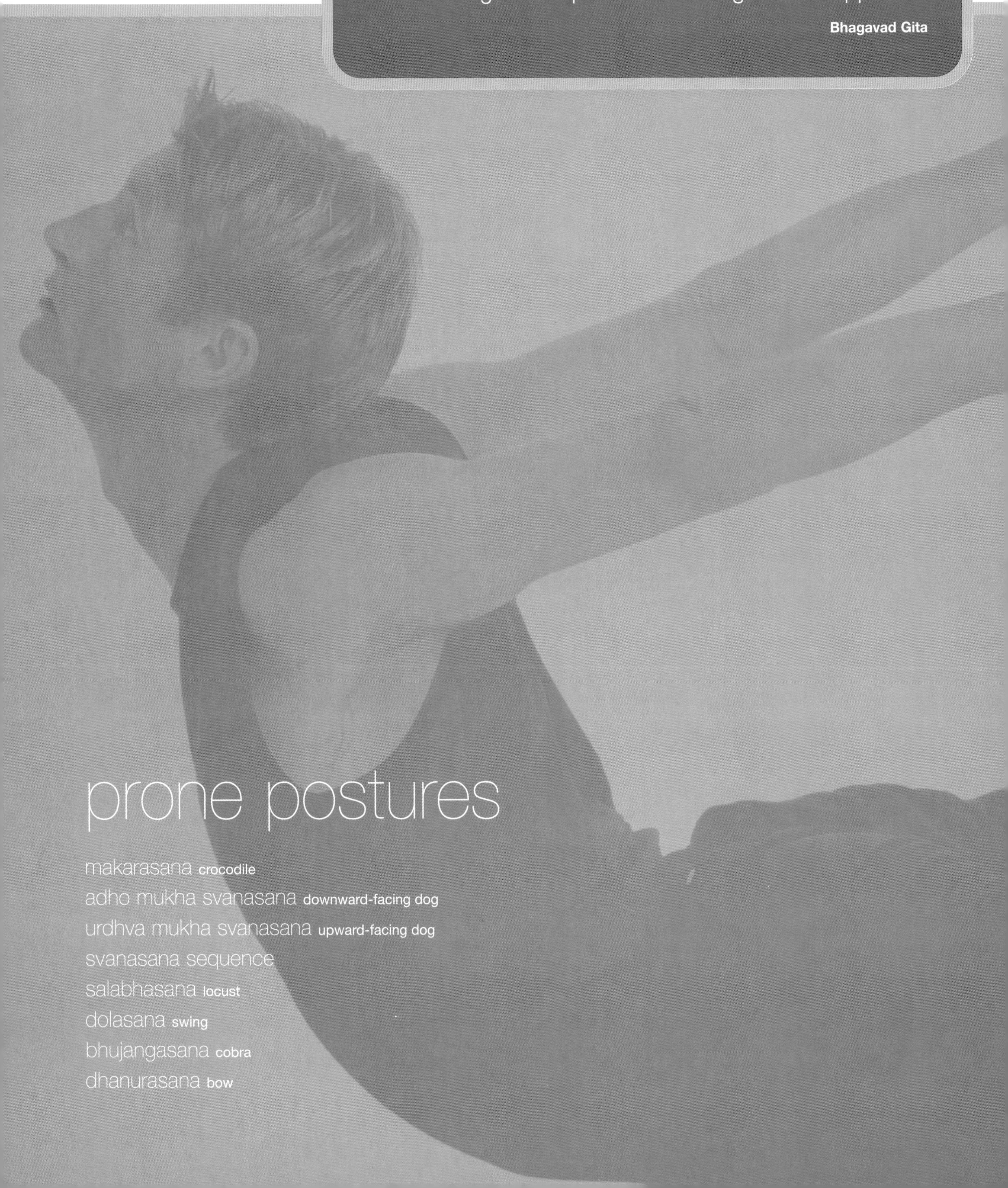

prone postures

makarasana crocodile

adho mukha svanasana downward-facing dog

urdhva mukha svanasana upward-facing dog

svanasana sequence

salabhasana locust

dolasana swing

bhujangasana cobra

dhanurasana bow

makarasana crocodile posture

Makara means "water creature" or "monster of the sea." Makarasana is a relaxation posture, which is useful for preparing for the rigorous prone postures. The arms and legs lie in full extension with all muscles supported by the floor.

level: Beginner

benefits • Rests the body and relieves fatigue • Quiets the mind

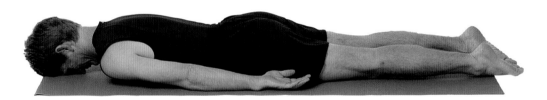

❶ Lie in a prone position, stretched out on a mat or a rug. Rest the forehead on the floor.

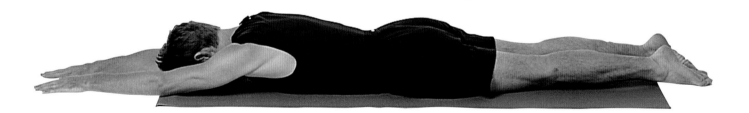

❷ Slowly stretch the arms out above the head. Turn the toes away from the body and lengthen the legs. Pull the shoulders, arms, and fingers forward. Now work on relaxing all the muscles, and feel the weight of your body supported by the floor.

adho mukha svanasana **downward-facing dog posture**

Adho means "downward," *mukha* means "face," and *svana* means "dog." This posture is based on the movements of a dog stretching downward. The spine and the legs are strongly stretched in this posture. Balasana (page 56) is a good posture to carry out before and after Svanasana.

level: Beginner

benefits • Strengthens and firms the back, neck, abdomen, and legs • Improves the circulation • Restores energy • Tones the reproductive organs

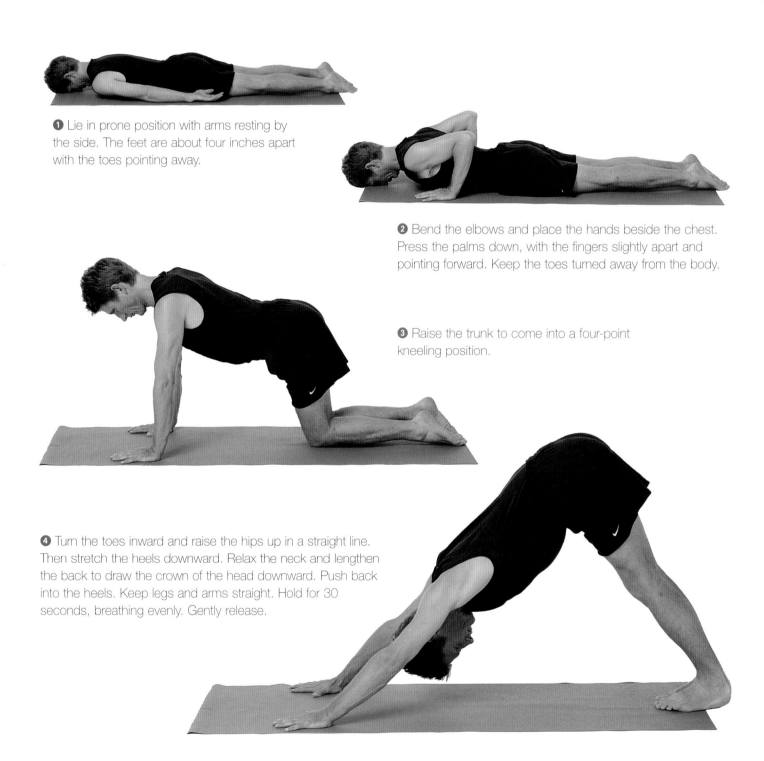

❶ Lie in prone position with arms resting by the side. The feet are about four inches apart with the toes pointing away.

❷ Bend the elbows and place the hands beside the chest. Press the palms down, with the fingers slightly apart and pointing forward. Keep the toes turned away from the body.

❸ Raise the trunk to come into a four-point kneeling position.

❹ Turn the toes inward and raise the hips up in a straight line. Then stretch the heels downward. Relax the neck and lengthen the back to draw the crown of the head downward. Push back into the heels. Keep legs and arms straight. Hold for 30 seconds, breathing evenly. Gently release.

urdhva mukha svanasana **upward-facing dog posture**

Urdhva means "upward," *mukha* means "face," and *svana* means "dog." This posture gives a vigorous upward stretch to the spine and counterstretches the downward movement of the Adho mukha svanasana. Balasana (page 56) is a good posture to carry out before and after Svanasana.

level: Beginner/Intermediate

caution: • This posture is not recommended if you have a weak back or wrists, or neck stiffness.

benefits • Strengthens the arms, legs, shoulders, and back • Improves the circulation • Invigorates the body

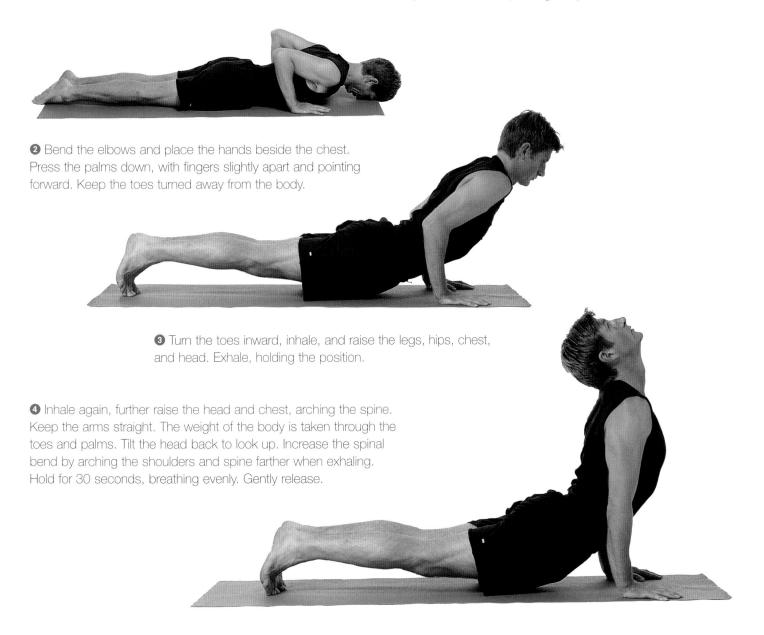

❶ Lie in a prone position with the arms resting by the side. The feet are about four inches apart with the toes pointing away.

❷ Bend the elbows and place the hands beside the chest. Press the palms down, with fingers slightly apart and pointing forward. Keep the toes turned away from the body.

❸ Turn the toes inward, inhale, and raise the legs, hips, chest, and head. Exhale, holding the position.

❹ Inhale again, further raise the head and chest, arching the spine. Keep the arms straight. The weight of the body is taken through the toes and palms. Tilt the head back to look up. Increase the spinal bend by arching the shoulders and spine farther when exhaling. Hold for 30 seconds, breathing evenly. Gently release.

svanasana sequence **dog sequence**

This sequence involves interchanging between Adho mukha svanasana and Urdhva mukha svanasana. The sequence gives a rigorous stretch to the spine. Before attempting this sequence, learn to hold the two positions of Svanasana for 10 minutes.

level: Intermediate/Advanced

caution: Strong arms, shoulders, and back are necessary for this sequence.

benefits • Strengthens and firms the back, neck, abdomen, and legs • Improves the circulation • Invigorates the body

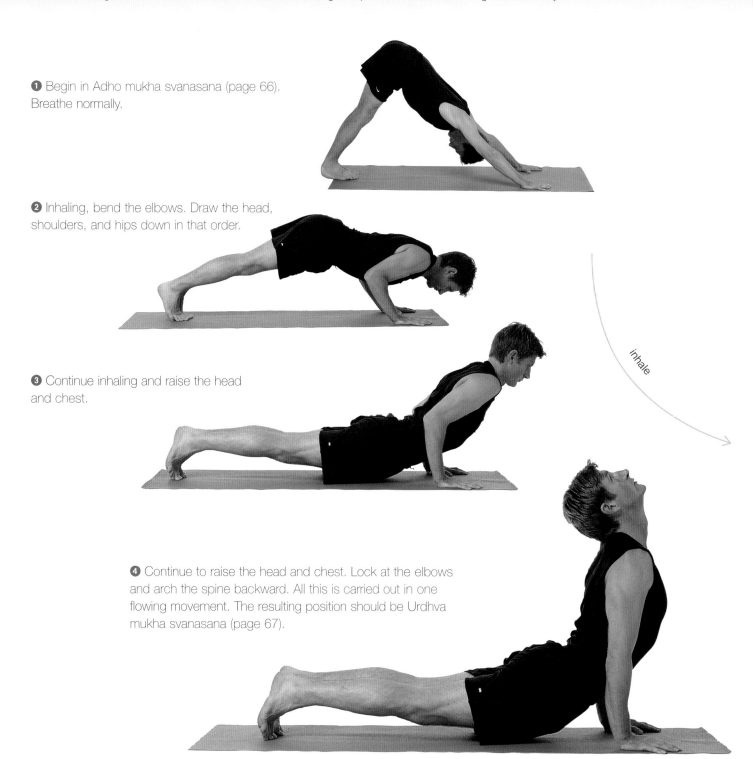

❶ Begin in Adho mukha svanasana (page 66). Breathe normally.

❷ Inhaling, bend the elbows. Draw the head, shoulders, and hips down in that order.

❸ Continue inhaling and raise the head and chest.

inhale

❹ Continue to raise the head and chest. Lock at the elbows and arch the spine backward. All this is carried out in one flowing movement. The resulting position should be Urdhva mukha svanasana (page 67).

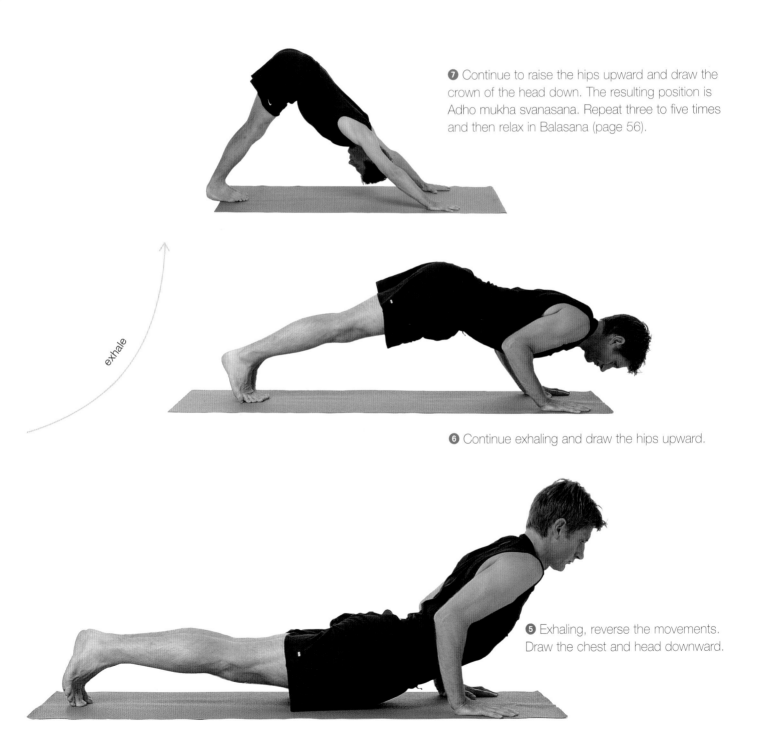

7 Continue to raise the hips upward and draw the crown of the head down. The resulting position is Adho mukha svanasana. Repeat three to five times and then relax in Balasana (page 56).

exhale

6 Continue exhaling and draw the hips upward.

5 Exhaling, reverse the movements. Draw the chest and head downward.

salabhasana locust posture

Salabha means "locust." Salabhasana is based on the resting locust with legs raised. This posture gives a stretch to the legs, abdomen, and lower back. The full Salabhasana requires considerable muscular effort. If it is difficult to achieve, then select one of the variations.

level: Intermediate

benefits • Regulates the function of the intestines • Improves the function of the liver, pancreas, and kidneys • Improves circulation

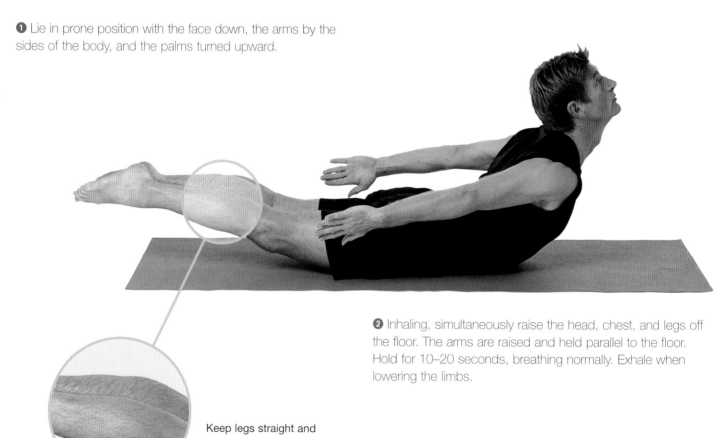

❶ Lie in prone position with the face down, the arms by the sides of the body, and the palms turned upward.

❷ Inhaling, simultaneously raise the head, chest, and legs off the floor. The arms are raised and held parallel to the floor. Hold for 10–20 seconds, breathing normally. Exhale when lowering the limbs.

Keep legs straight and close together.

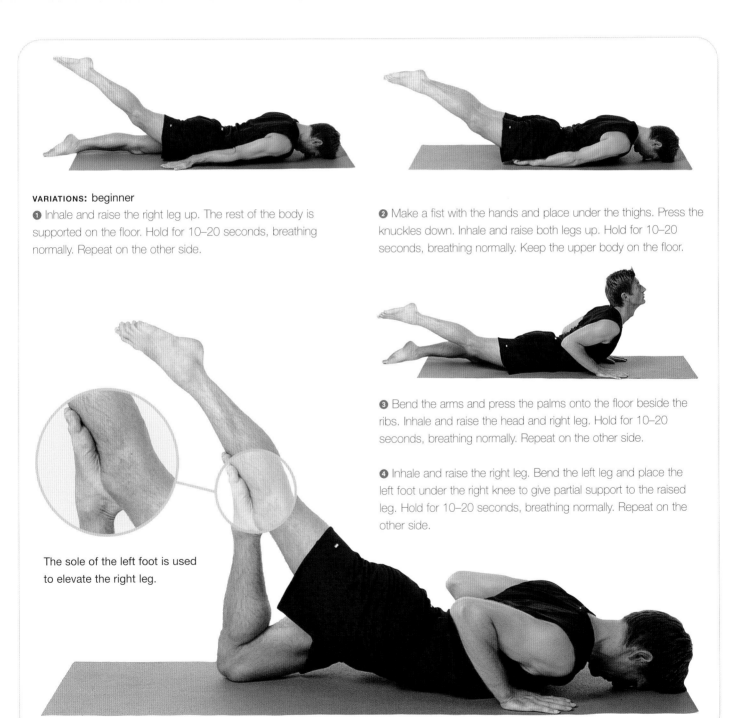

VARIATIONS: beginner

❶ Inhale and raise the right leg up. The rest of the body is supported on the floor. Hold for 10–20 seconds, breathing normally. Repeat on the other side.

❷ Make a fist with the hands and place under the thighs. Press the knuckles down. Inhale and raise both legs up. Hold for 10–20 seconds, breathing normally. Keep the upper body on the floor.

❸ Bend the arms and press the palms onto the floor beside the ribs. Inhale and raise the head and right leg. Hold for 10–20 seconds, breathing normally. Repeat on the other side.

❹ Inhale and raise the right leg. Bend the left leg and place the left foot under the right knee to give partial support to the raised leg. Hold for 10–20 seconds, breathing normally. Repeat on the other side.

The sole of the left foot is used to elevate the right leg.

dolasana swing posture

Dola means "swing." In Dolasana the spine is arched by raising the legs and arms. The shape of the body is like that of a hammock. It is a good posture to practice if Dhanurasana is difficult.

level: Beginner

benefits • Tones the abdomen, legs, and arms • Promotes agility in the body

❶ Lie in Makarasana (page 65).

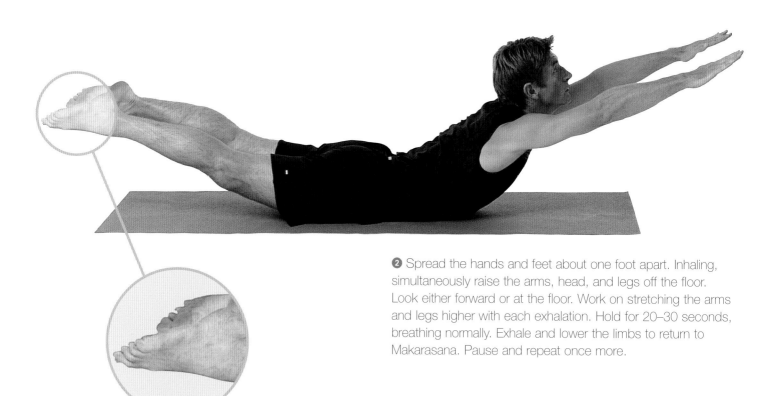

❷ Spread the hands and feet about one foot apart. Inhaling, simultaneously raise the arms, head, and legs off the floor. Look either forward or at the floor. Work on stretching the arms and legs higher with each exhalation. Hold for 20–30 seconds, breathing normally. Exhale and lower the limbs to return to Makarasana. Pause and repeat once more.

Point the toes away from the body.

bhujangasana **cobra posture**

Bhujanga means "cobra." Bhujangasana resembles the cobra with its crownlike head raised up regally. The lumbar spine is arched, resulting in the abdomen being strongly stretched. Balasana (page 56) is a useful counterstretch to the strong spinal bend of Bhujangasana.

level: Beginner/Intermediate

caution: This posture is not recommended for people with lower back problems.

benefits • Strengthens the back muscles • Improves the function of the digestive system • Regulates the menstrual flow

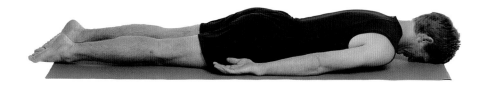

❶ Lie in a prone position with the legs together. Rest the forehead on the floor.

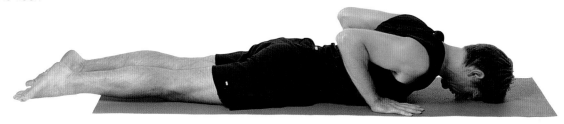

❷ Bend the arms and press the palms down under the shoulders.

Relax the hips and abdomen.

❸ Inhale as the head and chest are raised off the floor. Pause to exhale. Inhale again and continue to raise the head and chest farther. Tilt the head back and point the chin upward. Retain a slight bend in the elbows, keeping them close to the body. Draw the shoulders downward and relax the abdomen and legs. Work on arching the spine slightly more when exhaling. Hold for 20–30 seconds, breathing normally. Exhale while lowering the upper body back to the floor.

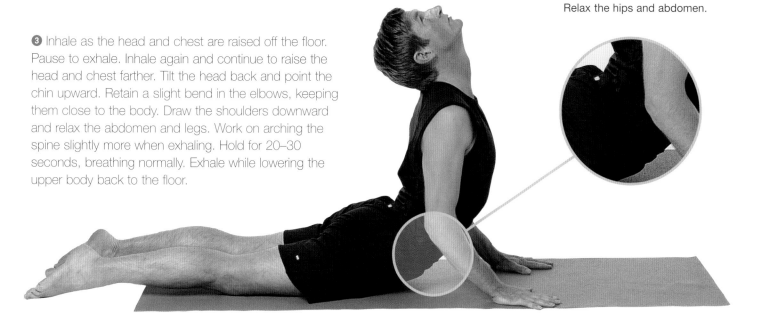

dhanurasana bow posture

Dhanura means "bow." In this posture the body assumes a bow shape. The arms are linked to the ankles and held taut like the string of a bow. Dhanurasana combines the effect of Bhujangasana (page 73) and Salabhasana (pages 70–71). Hence the spine is strongly arched and the whole weight of the body is on the solar plexus.

level: Intermediate/Advanced

caution: This is a rigorous posture and is not recommended for people with lower back problems.

benefits • Strengthens the spine • Massages the abdominal organs • Regulates the menstrual flow • Increases stamina • Promotes a stronger voice

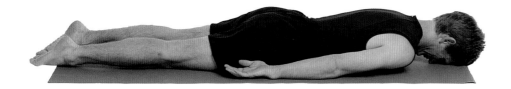

❶ Lie in a prone position with the arms beside the trunk and the forehead resting on the floor.

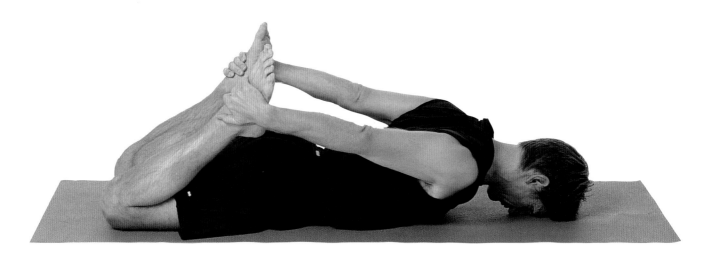

❷ Inhale, bend the legs back, and clasp the ankles firmly with the hands. If holding the ankles is difficult, then hold the feet.

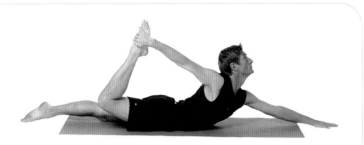

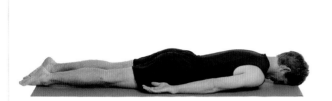

VARIATION: Beginner/Intermediate

In Ardha dhanurasana (Half-bow), one leg is raised at a time. Lie prone with the arms stretched in front. Fold the right leg back and clasp the ankle with the right hand. The left leg and arm are stretched straight. Inhale and raise the head, chest, and right thigh off the floor. Hold for 10–20 seconds, breathing evenly. Release and repeat on the other side.

❸ Inhale and simultaneously raise the head, chest, and thighs off the floor. If it is uncomfortable to raise the thighs, then keep them on the floor and press the heels into the thighs. Breathe deeply and evenly, holding for 20 seconds. Exhale to release the hold on the legs and rest the limbs and body on the floor. Finish with Balasana (page 56).

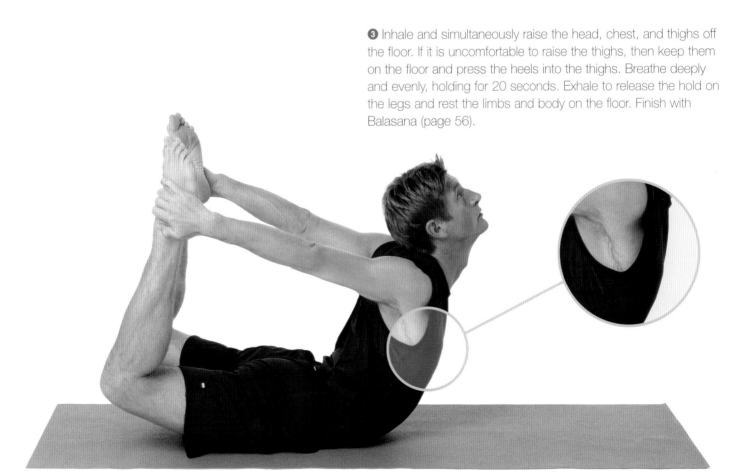

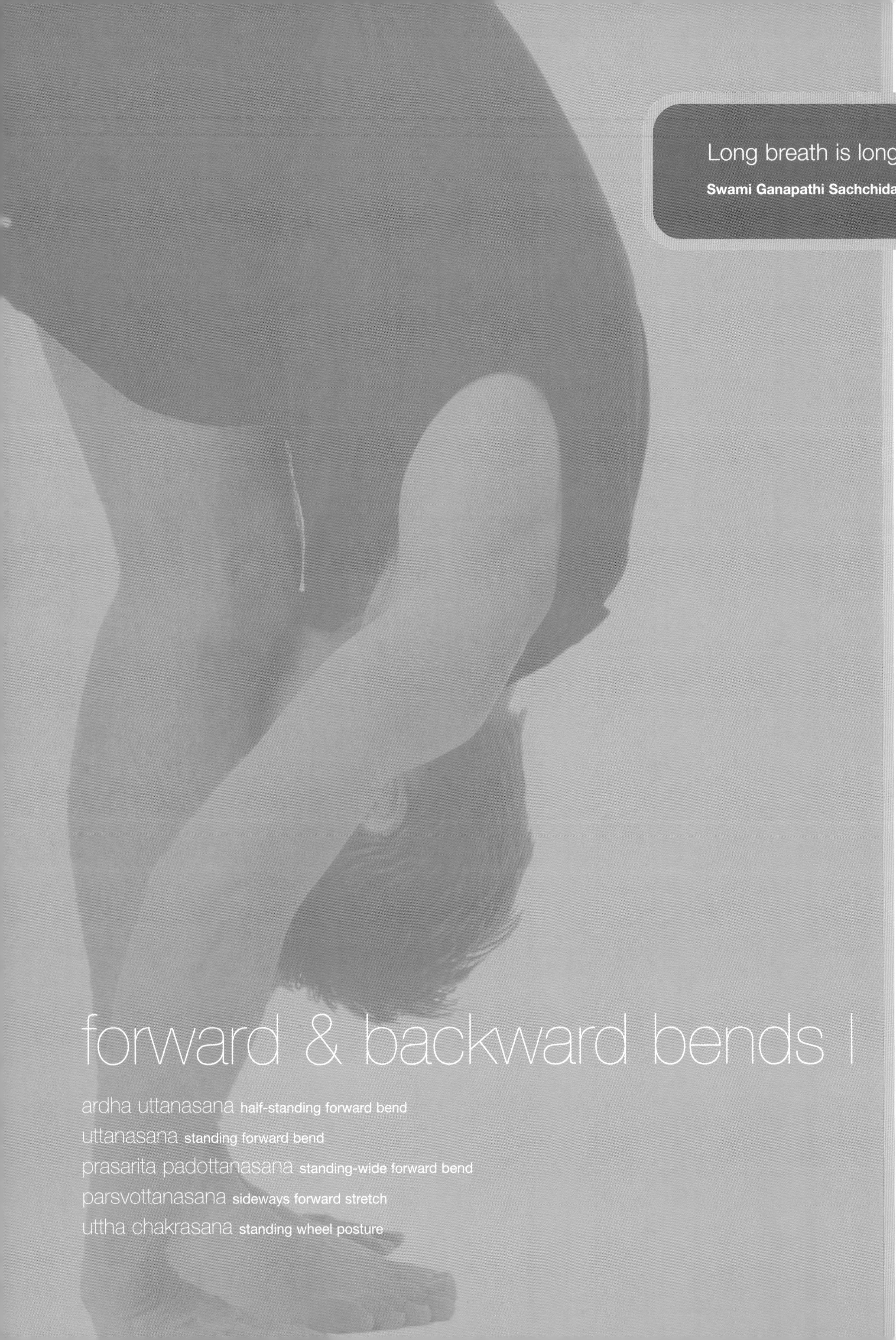

Long breath is long life.

Swami Ganapathi Sachchidananda

forward & backward bends I

ardha uttanasana half-standing forward bend

uttanasana standing forward bend

prasarita padottanasana standing-wide forward bend

parsvottanasana sideways forward stretch

uttha chakrasana standing wheel posture

ardha uttanasana **half-standing forward bend**

Ardha means "half" and *uttana* means "extension." This position is especially useful if you cannot place the fingers or palms on the floor in the forward bend. Use it as an alternative to or in preparation for Uttanasana (page 78).

level: Beginner

caution: Avoid curving the back, as this can reinforce back stiffness or pain.

benefits • Relieves back pain • Strengthens the wrist and ankles • Calms the mind

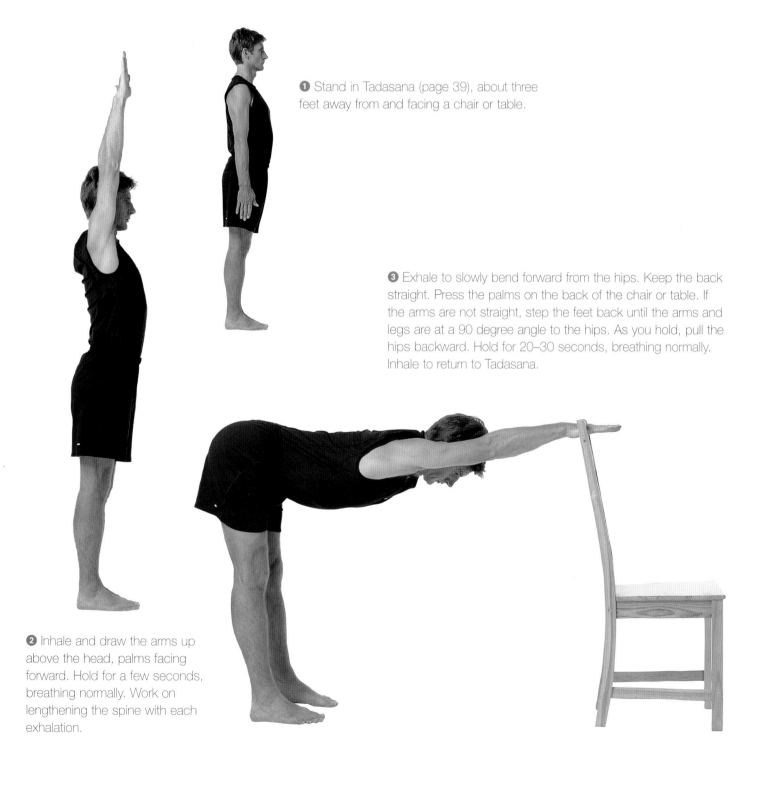

❶ Stand in Tadasana (page 39), about three feet away from and facing a chair or table.

❸ Exhale to slowly bend forward from the hips. Keep the back straight. Press the palms on the back of the chair or table. If the arms are not straight, step the feet back until the arms and legs are at a 90 degree angle to the hips. As you hold, pull the hips backward. Hold for 20–30 seconds, breathing normally. Inhale to return to Tadasana.

❷ Inhale and draw the arms up above the head, palms facing forward. Hold for a few seconds, breathing normally. Work on lengthening the spine with each exhalation.

uttanasana **standing forward bend**

Uttana means "extension." In Uttanasana the upper body is bent forward, allowing the spine and legs to be lengthened and extensively stretched. It is a useful posture to follow the strenuous standing postures and prepare for Paschimottanasana (page 87).

level: Beginner

caution: Not suitable for individuals with a slipped disk.

benefits • Refreshes the mind • Rejuvenates the nervous system • Relieves menstrual discomfort • Has a beneficial effect on the liver and spleen

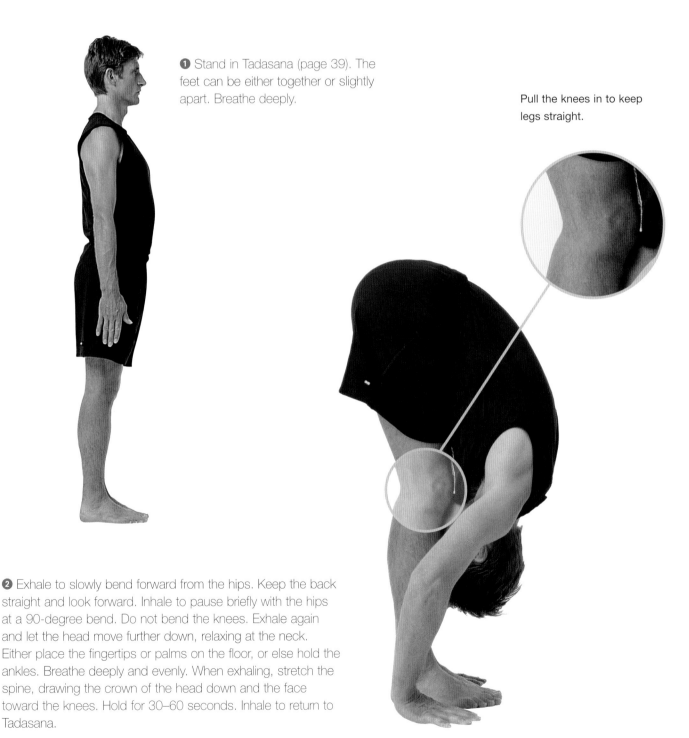

❶ Stand in Tadasana (page 39). The feet can be either together or slightly apart. Breathe deeply.

Pull the knees in to keep legs straight.

❷ Exhale to slowly bend forward from the hips. Keep the back straight and look forward. Inhale to pause briefly with the hips at a 90-degree bend. Do not bend the knees. Exhale again and let the head move further down, relaxing at the neck. Either place the fingertips or palms on the floor, or else hold the ankles. Breathe deeply and evenly. When exhaling, stretch the spine, drawing the crown of the head down and the face toward the knees. Hold for 30–60 seconds. Inhale to return to Tadasana.

prasarita padottanasana **standing-wide forward bend**

Prasarita means "spread wide." *Pada* means "foot" or "leg." Prasarita padottanasana stretches the hamstrings and widens the groin. The arches of the feet are pulled up and the blood flow to the chest and heart is increased. This is a good alternative to Sirshasana (page 122).

level: Beginner

caution: If the full forward bend is uncomfortable, then practice bending 90 degrees with palms placed on a table or chair.

benefits • Tones the legs • Improves circulation • Invigorates the mind

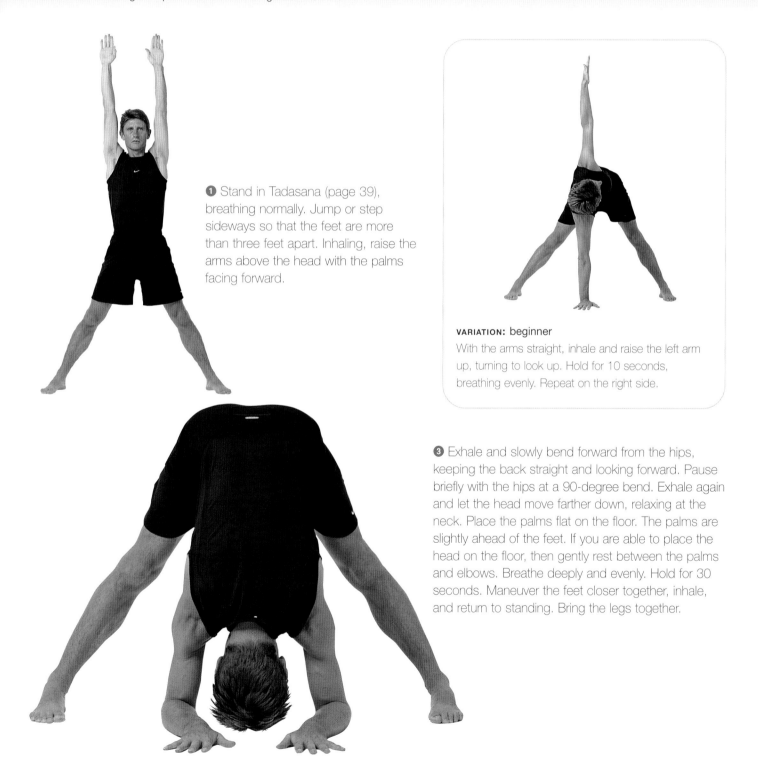

❶ Stand in Tadasana (page 39), breathing normally. Jump or step sideways so that the feet are more than three feet apart. Inhaling, raise the arms above the head with the palms facing forward.

VARIATION: beginner

With the arms straight, inhale and raise the left arm up, turning to look up. Hold for 10 seconds, breathing evenly. Repeat on the right side.

❸ Exhale and slowly bend forward from the hips, keeping the back straight and looking forward. Pause briefly with the hips at a 90-degree bend. Exhale again and let the head move farther down, relaxing at the neck. Place the palms flat on the floor. The palms are slightly ahead of the feet. If you are able to place the head on the floor, then gently rest between the palms and elbows. Breathe deeply and evenly. Hold for 30 seconds. Maneuver the feet closer together, inhale, and return to standing. Bring the legs together.

parsvottanasana sideways forward stretch

Parsva means "sideways" and *uttana* means "extension." In Parsvottanasana, the chest is expanded as the shoulders are pulled back with the hand position. It corrects rounded shoulders and increases awareness of posture.

level: Intermediate

caution: If the prayer position is uncomfortable, link the hands to the opposite forearms.

benefits • Improves posture and balance • Increases the flexibility of the wrists, hips, and spine • Deepens the breath and cleanses the lungs

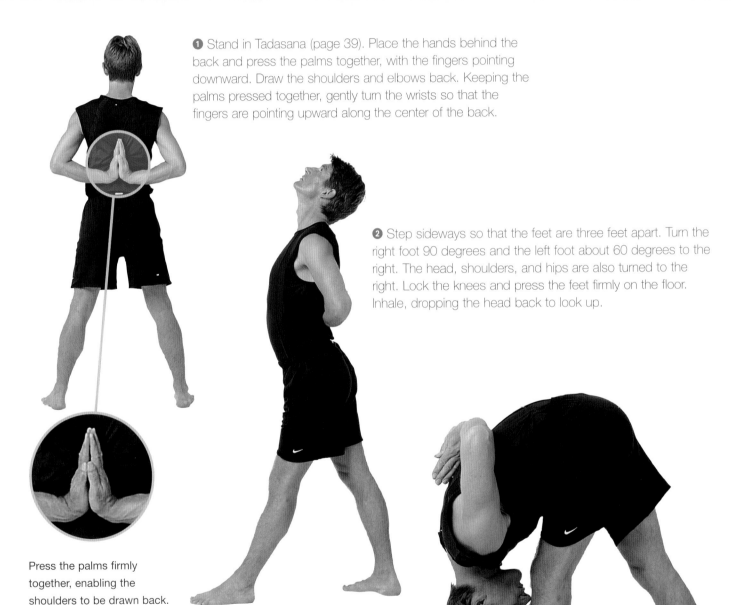

❶ Stand in Tadasana (page 39). Place the hands behind the back and press the palms together, with the fingers pointing downward. Draw the shoulders and elbows back. Keeping the palms pressed together, gently turn the wrists so that the fingers are pointing upward along the center of the back.

❷ Step sideways so that the feet are three feet apart. Turn the right foot 90 degrees and the left foot about 60 degrees to the right. The head, shoulders, and hips are also turned to the right. Lock the knees and press the feet firmly on the floor. Inhale, dropping the head back to look up.

Press the palms firmly together, enabling the shoulders to be drawn back.

❸ Exhale, bending forward slowly from the hips. Relaxing at the neck, let the crown of the head move downward and the face toward the knee. Hold for 20 seconds, breathing normally. Inhale to return to standing. Repeat, bending toward the left. Repeat again, but with the feet facing forward and bending to the center.

uttha chakrasana **standing wheel posture**

Uttha means "standing" and *chakra* means "wheel" or "energy vortex." In Utta chakrasana the back is arched, stretching the lumbar and thoracic spine. The legs and hips are held firm to enable the bend. Move slowly into the stretch to avoid disorientation. This posture is often seen to be a variation of Chakrasana (page 98).

level: Beginner

caution: If prone to dizziness or stiffness in the neck or lower back, avoid this stretch. Instead, hold for longer in the Uttanasana (page 78).

benefits • Deepens the breath • Increases flexibility of the spine • Energizes tired muscles

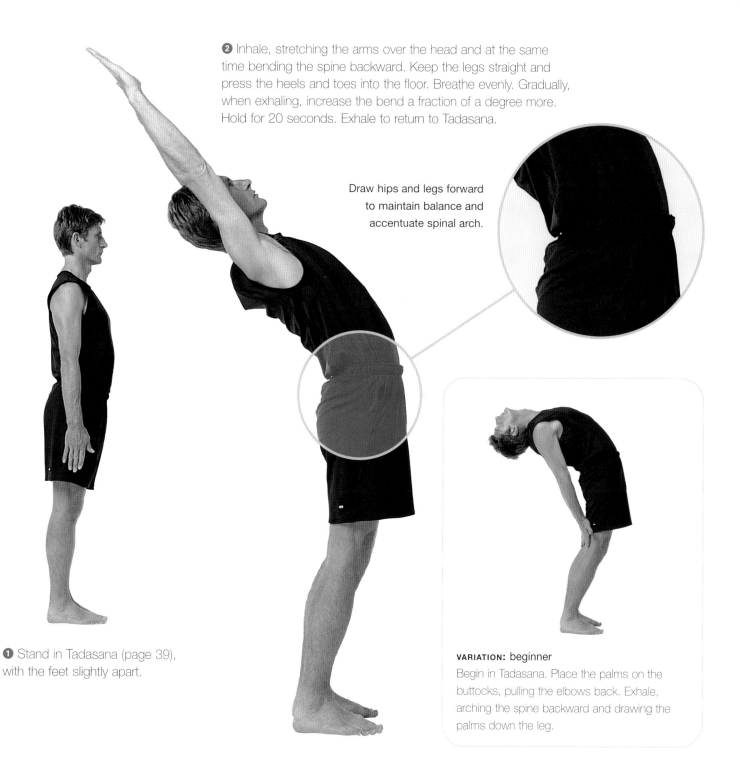

❷ Inhale, stretching the arms over the head and at the same time bending the spine backward. Keep the legs straight and press the heels and toes into the floor. Breathe evenly. Gradually, when exhaling, increase the bend a fraction of a degree more. Hold for 20 seconds. Exhale to return to Tadasana.

Draw hips and legs forward to maintain balance and accentuate spinal arch.

❶ Stand in Tadasana (page 39), with the feet slightly apart.

VARIATION: beginner
Begin in Tadasana. Place the palms on the buttocks, pulling the elbows back. Exhale, arching the spine backward and drawing the palms down the leg.

One should practice the asanas, which give the yogi strength, keep him in good health, and make his limbs supple.

Hatha Yoga Pradipika

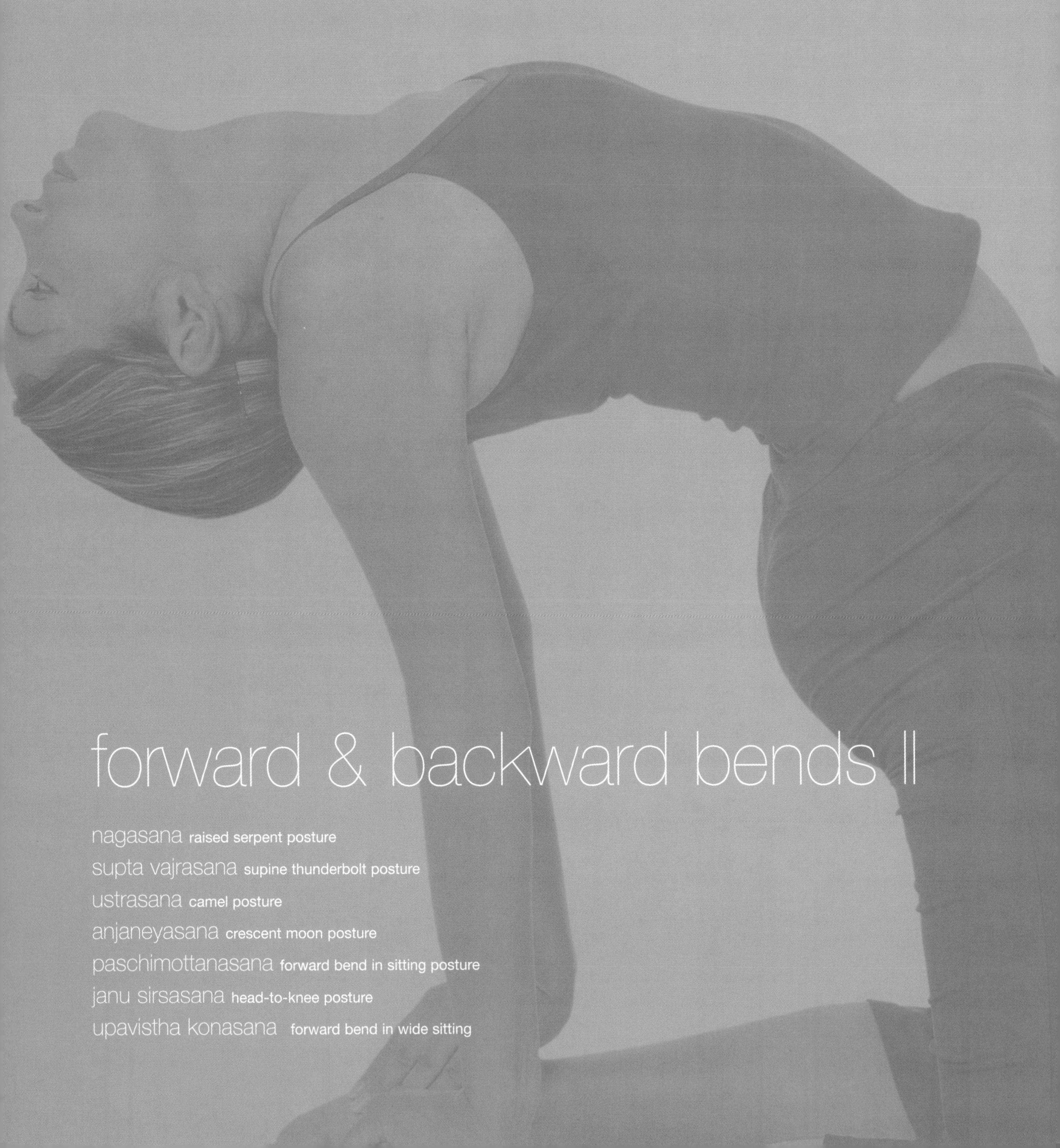

forward & backward bends II

nagasana raised serpent posture

supta vajrasana supine thunderbolt posture

ustrasana camel posture

anjaneyasana crescent moon posture

paschimottanasana forward bend in sitting posture

janu sirsasana head-to-knee posture

upavistha konasana forward bend in wide sitting

nagasana raised serpent posture

Naga means "snake." Nagasana is based on the flowing movements of the snake. As the arms and head are drawn backward, the lumbar and thoracic spine are stretched. The kneeling position has a wider base of support, allowing the body to arch back.

level: Beginner

caution: Avoid if prone to lower back problems.

benefits • Strengthens the knees, ankles, and spine • Deepens the breath • Improves posture and balance • Strengthens the wrists and ankles

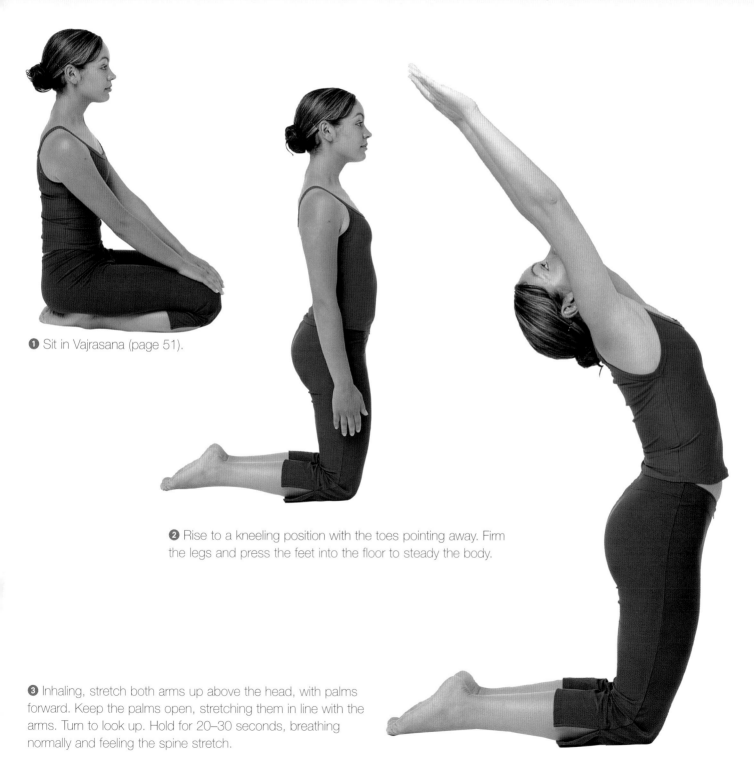

❶ Sit in Vajrasana (page 51).

❷ Rise to a kneeling position with the toes pointing away. Firm the legs and press the feet into the floor to steady the body.

❸ Inhaling, stretch both arms up above the head, with palms forward. Keep the palms open, stretching them in line with the arms. Turn to look up. Hold for 20–30 seconds, breathing normally and feeling the spine stretch.

supta vajrasana supine thunderbolt posture

Supta means "resting" or "sleeping" and *Vajra* means "thunderbolt." In Supta vajrasana, the trunk is reclined backward. This is a difficult stretch to achieve; the beginner should first practice the variation shown below. Balasana (page 56) is a good counterstretch to this posture.

level: Intermediate/Advanced

caution: If you have a back problem, consult your doctor before practicing strong backward stretches.

benefits • Massages the abdominal organs and the pelvic region • Aids digestion, as it can be practiced after a meal • Relieves tired legs

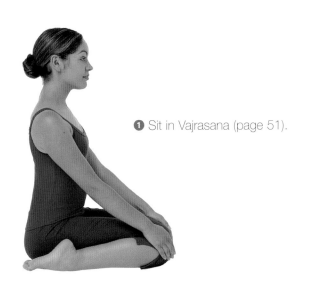

❶ Sit in Vajrasana (page 51).

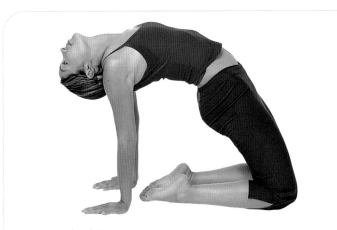

VARIATION: beginner
Lean back and place the hands to the rear with the fingers pointing away. Inhale, slowly raising the pelvis and trunk and tilting the head back. Work on drawing the pelvis upward. Breathe normally.

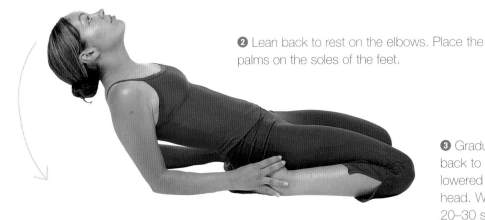

❷ Lean back to rest on the elbows. Place the palms on the soles of the feet.

❸ Gradually bring the back of the head and the back to rest on the floor. The entire body is lowered onto the floor. Stretch the arms over the head. Work on relaxing the back muscles. Hold for 20–30 seconds, breathing deeply. To return to Vajrasana, reverse the body movements used to go into the stretch.

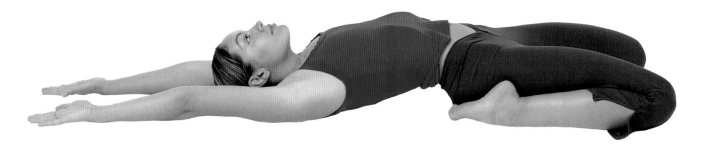

ustrasana camel posture

Ustra means "camel." In Ustrasana the whole body is stretched and the chest is expanded as the arms and shoulders are pulled back. Beginners should first practice the variation shown below.

level: Intermediate

caution: If this posture is uncomfortable, practice the Paschimottanasana (page 87) for a longer period.

benefits • Cleanses the lungs • Improves circulation • Improves function of the thyroid gland and reproductive organs • Corrects rounded shoulders

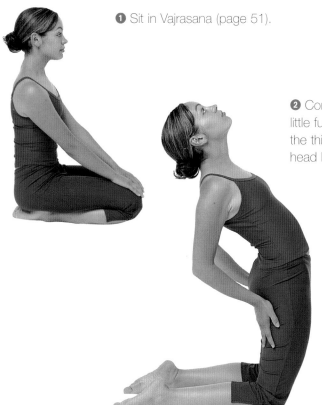

❶ Sit in Vajrasana (page 51).

❷ Come to a kneeling position and take the knees and feet a little further apart. Place the hands on the hips. Inhale, press the thighs and hips forward and arch the spine back. Tilt the head back to look up. Exhale.

❸ Inhale again to bend the spine farther and stretch the hands back to rest on the heels. Tilt the head back farther. Focus on pressing the hips forward and increasing the arch of the spine while keeping the thighs vertical. Hold for 10–20 seconds, breathing normally. Inhale to gently release.

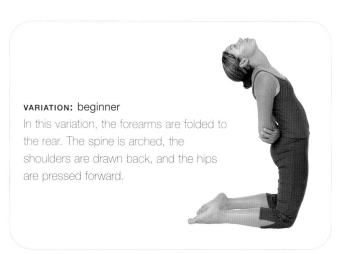

VARIATION: beginner
In this variation, the forearms are folded to the rear. The spine is arched, the shoulders are drawn back, and the hips are pressed forward.

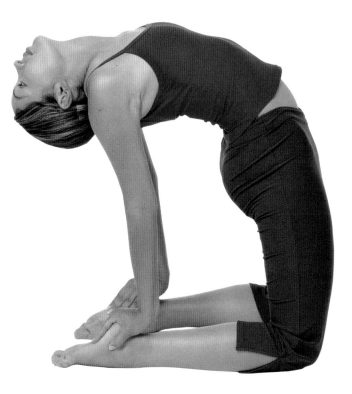

anjaneyasana **crescent moon posture**

Anja means "form" and *neya* means "reduced" or "time passed." In Anjaneyasana, the spine is strongly arched and the rear leg is stretched. The entire body makes an arc, resembling the shape of the crescent moon.

level: Intermediate

caution: If prone to back problems, consult a doctor before practicing strong backward stretches.

benefits • Regulates the digestive system • Strengthens the ankles and legs

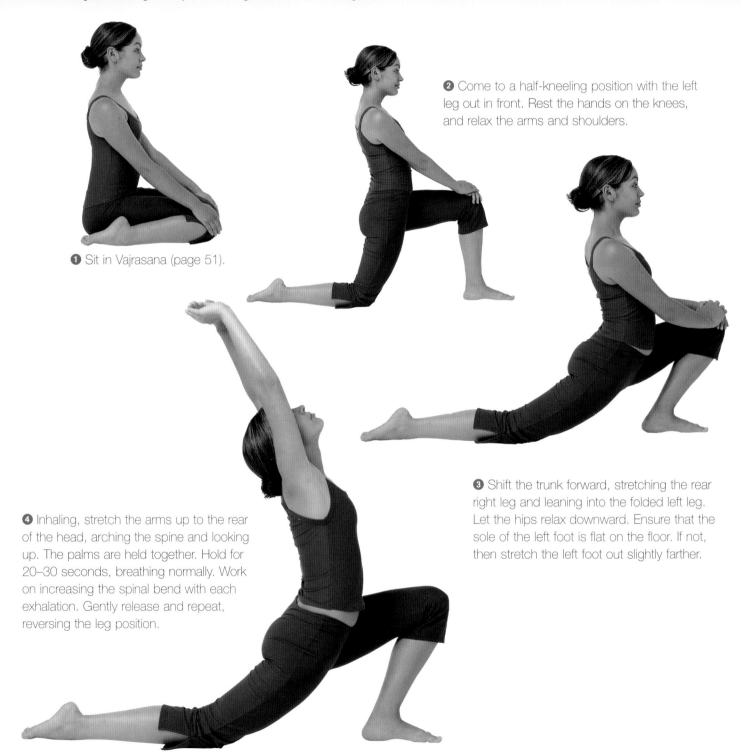

❶ Sit in Vajrasana (page 51).

❷ Come to a half-kneeling position with the left leg out in front. Rest the hands on the knees, and relax the arms and shoulders.

❸ Shift the trunk forward, stretching the rear right leg and leaning into the folded left leg. Let the hips relax downward. Ensure that the sole of the left foot is flat on the floor. If not, then stretch the left foot out slightly farther.

❹ Inhaling, stretch the arms up to the rear of the head, arching the spine and looking up. The palms are held together. Hold for 20–30 seconds, breathing normally. Work on increasing the spinal bend with each exhalation. Gently release and repeat, reversing the leg position.

paschimottanasana **forward bend in sitting**

Paschima means "back" and *uttana* means "extension." In Paschimottanasana, the whole body is stretched. The respiratory rate is said to be reduced by 50 percent. It is widely regarded as one of the most important postures in yoga. Regular practice is needed to master this stretch.

level: Beginner

caution: If discomfort is experienced in the abdomen, reduce the bend to ease the pressure on the abdomen.

benefits • Improves the digestive system and abdominal organs • Soothes and refreshes the mind • Develops patience

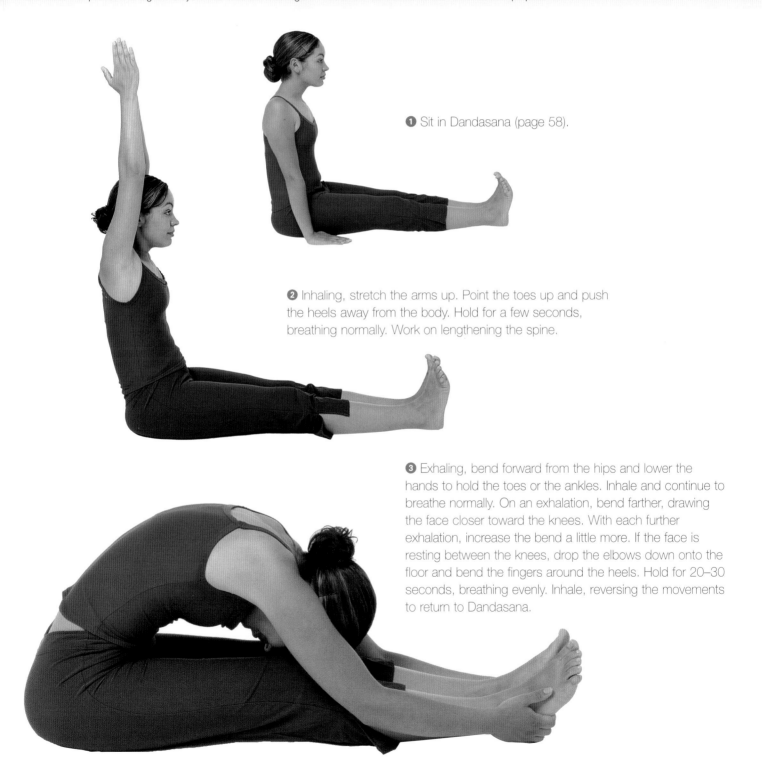

❶ Sit in Dandasana (page 58).

❷ Inhaling, stretch the arms up. Point the toes up and push the heels away from the body. Hold for a few seconds, breathing normally. Work on lengthening the spine.

❸ Exhaling, bend forward from the hips and lower the hands to hold the toes or the ankles. Inhale and continue to breathe normally. On an exhalation, bend farther, drawing the face closer toward the knees. With each further exhalation, increase the bend a little more. If the face is resting between the knees, drop the elbows down onto the floor and bend the fingers around the heels. Hold for 20–30 seconds, breathing evenly. Inhale, reversing the movements to return to Dandasana.

janu sirsasana head-to-knee posture

Janu means "knee" and *sirsa* means "head." In Janu sirsasana the bent leg gives a good anchor to the body and assists the forward bend toward the straight leg.

level: Beginner

benefits • Tones the kidneys • Regulates the digestive system • Strengthens the ankles and legs

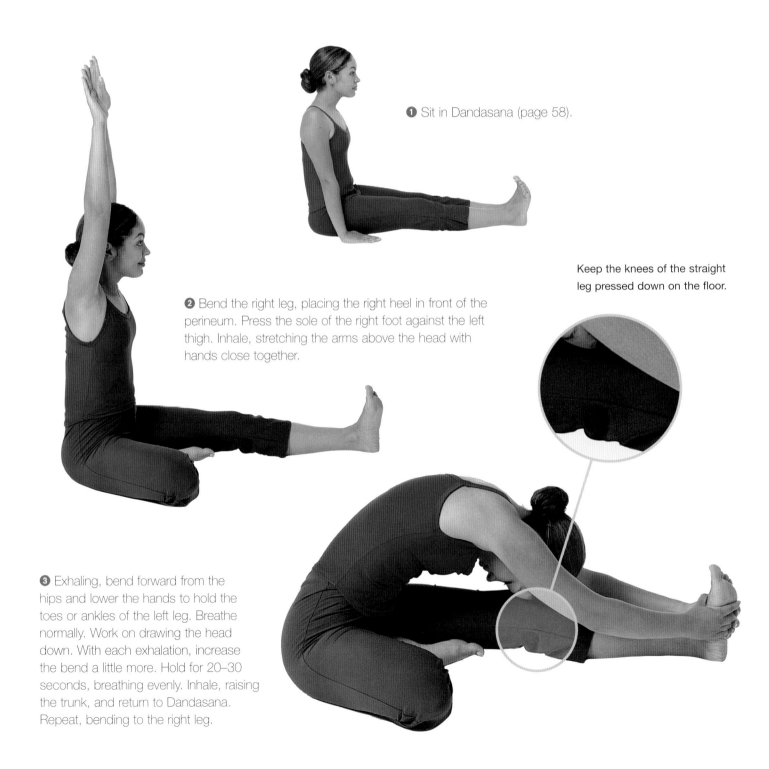

❶ Sit in Dandasana (page 58).

Keep the knees of the straight leg pressed down on the floor.

❷ Bend the right leg, placing the right heel in front of the perineum. Press the sole of the right foot against the left thigh. Inhale, stretching the arms above the head with hands close together.

❸ Exhaling, bend forward from the hips and lower the hands to hold the toes or ankles of the left leg. Breathe normally. Work on drawing the head down. With each exhalation, increase the bend a little more. Hold for 20–30 seconds, breathing evenly. Inhale, raising the trunk, and return to Dandasana. Repeat, bending to the right leg.

upavistha konasana forward bend in wide sitting

Upavistha means "seated" and *kona* means "angle." Upavistha konasana is another sitting forward bend posture. The legs are stretched at a wide angle and the upper body is bent forward.

level: Beginner/Intermediate

caution: Do not overstretch the neck when drawing the head closer to the floor. If stretching the hamstrings is uncomfortable, place the hands farther on the ankle.

benefits • Tones the legs • Massages the abdominal organs

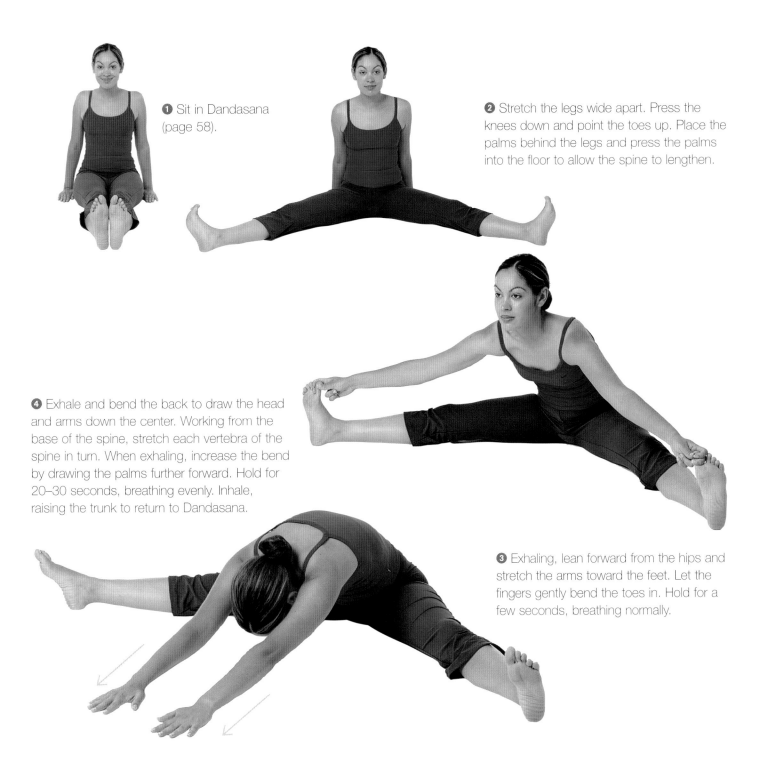

❶ Sit in Dandasana (page 58).

❷ Stretch the legs wide apart. Press the knees down and point the toes up. Place the palms behind the legs and press the palms into the floor to allow the spine to lengthen.

❹ Exhale and bend the back to draw the head and arms down the center. Working from the base of the spine, stretch each vertebra of the spine in turn. When exhaling, increase the bend by drawing the palms further forward. Hold for 20–30 seconds, breathing evenly. Inhale, raising the trunk to return to Dandasana.

❸ Exhaling, lean forward from the hips and stretch the arms toward the feet. Let the fingers gently bend the toes in. Hold for a few seconds, breathing normally.

Asanas make one firm, free from maladies, and light of limb.

Hatha Yoga Pradipika

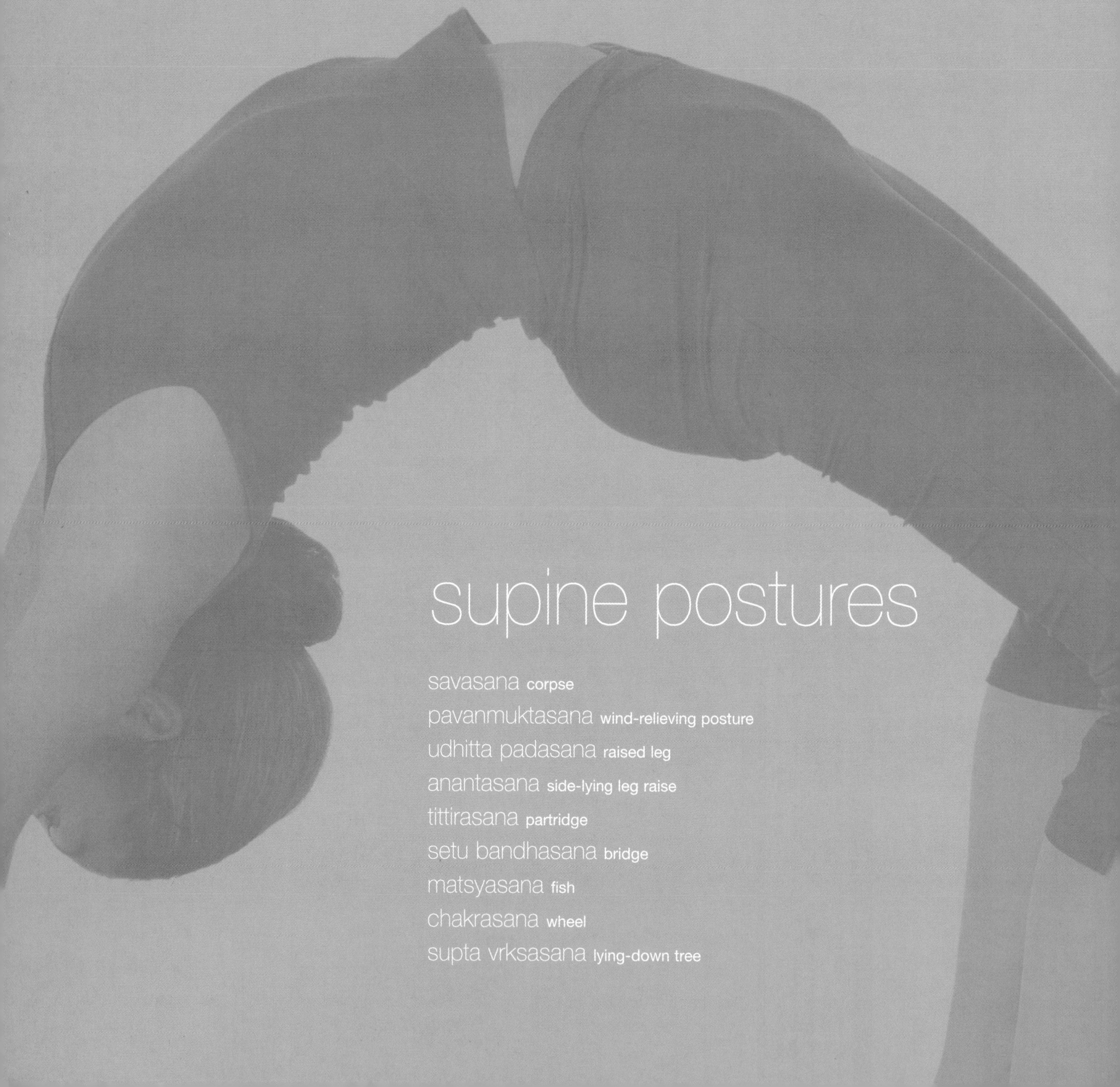

supine postures

savasana corpse

pavanmuktasana wind-relieving posture

udhitta padasana raised leg

anantasana side-lying leg raise

tittirasana partridge

setu bandhasana bridge

matsyasana fish

chakrasana wheel

supta vrksasana lying-down tree

savasana corpse posture

Sava means "corpse." In Savasana the body lies still, with the muscles completely relaxed. Mental activity is reduced to a minimum and the breath is deepened. The body senses are withdrawn from the surroundings. Spending ten minutes in Savasana is said to lower the blood pressure and bring rest equivalent to that derived from a night's sleep.

level: Beginner

benefits • Refreshes the mind and body • Lowers the blood pressure

❶ Lie in a supine position. Adjust the body to ensure that the head is positioned in the center and the spine feels aligned. The arms are slightly away from the body and the legs are slightly apart. The palms are turned upward and the fingers are curled up as tension is released. Close the eyes and focus on the breath. With each exhalation, release the tension and tightness in all the muscles. Let the breath flow in and out effortlessly.

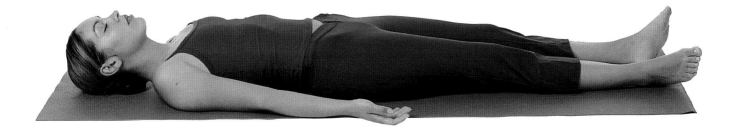

pavanmuktasana wind-relieving posture

Pavan means "wind" and *mukta* means "liberated." Pavanmuktasana is a relaxing posture, which is akin to Balasana (page 56). It is an excellent counterstretch to the strong spinal bends. A rocking motion carried out in this posture helps to release tension in the back muscles.

level: Beginner

benefits • Releases intestinal gas • Limbers up the spine, hips, and legs • Cleanses the lungs

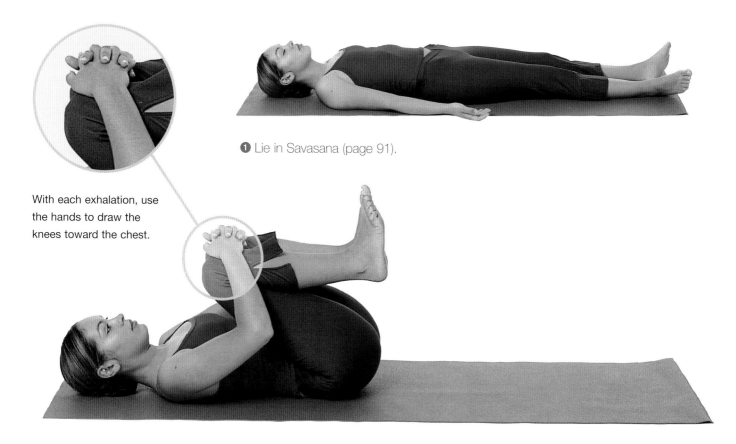

❶ Lie in Savasana (page 91).

With each exhalation, use the hands to draw the knees toward the chest.

❷ Exhale and draw the knees to the chest. Clasp the hands over the knees and use them to compress the knees closer to the chest. Inhale and exhale again; with the inhalation, decrease the pressure, and with the exhalation, increase the pressure. Continue for 30–60 seconds. Release to stretch the legs back onto the floor.

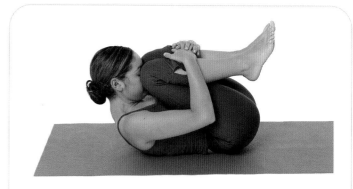

VARIATION: beginner
Raise both legs and raise the head to draw the forehead to the knees.

udhitta padasana **raised leg posture**

Udhitta means "raise" and *pada* means "leg" or "foot." Udhitta padasana develops the stomach muscles needed to carry out more advanced supine postures.

level: Beginner

caution: If prone to lower back problems, avoid the double leg raise. Instead practice the single leg raise at first.

benefits • Tones the legs and abdomen • Strengthens the stomach muscles

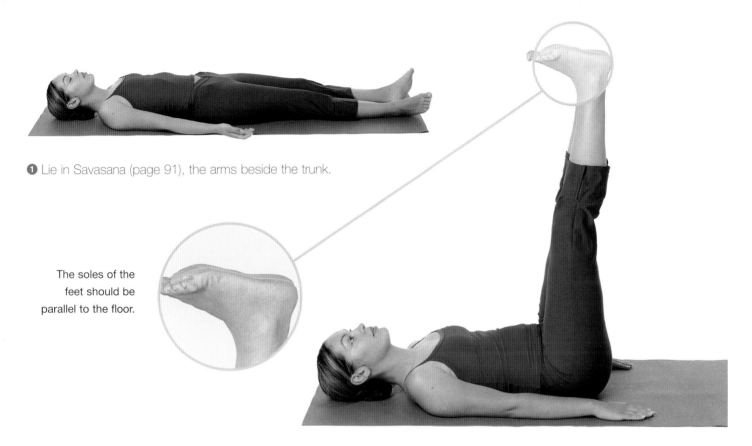

❶ Lie in Savasana (page 91), the arms beside the trunk.

The soles of the feet should be parallel to the floor.

❷ Exhale and raise both the legs 90 degrees. The legs are straight, with the knee muscles pulled tight. Turn the toes in and push the heels up. Hold for 30 seconds, breathing naturally. Gently lower the legs to the floor to release. Repeat once more.

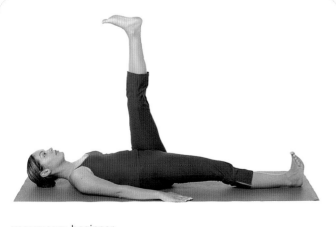

VARIATIONS: beginner

❶ Raise one leg at a time.

❷ Raise both legs and use the wall for support.

anantasana side-lying leg raise

Ananta means "without end" or "eternity." Like the previous posture, Anantasana stretches and tones the legs. This posture is particularly beneficial for cyclists and runners.

level: Beginner

benefits • Stretches the hamstrings • Limbers up the hips • Strengthens the wrists

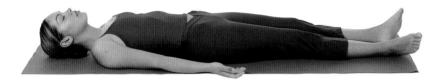

❶ Lie in Savasana (page 91), with the arms beside the trunk.

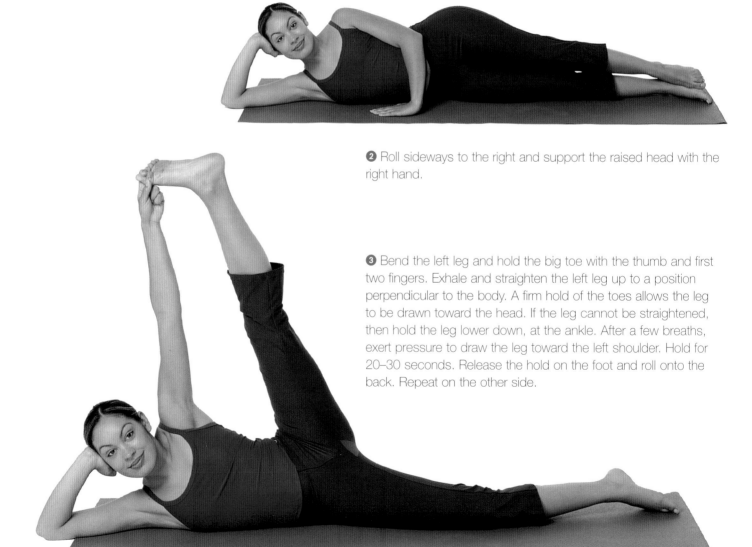

❷ Roll sideways to the right and support the raised head with the right hand.

❸ Bend the left leg and hold the big toe with the thumb and first two fingers. Exhale and straighten the left leg up to a position perpendicular to the body. A firm hold of the toes allows the leg to be drawn toward the head. If the leg cannot be straightened, then hold the leg lower down, at the ankle. After a few breaths, exert pressure to draw the leg toward the left shoulder. Hold for 20–30 seconds. Release the hold on the foot and roll onto the back. Repeat on the other side.

tittirasana partridge posture

Tittiri means "partridge." Tittirasana is based on the unusual sleeping position of the tittiri, which slumbers with its legs raised up in the air. In this posture, the legs are stretched up wide from a supine position.

level: Beginner

benefits • Tones the legs and arms • Limbers up the pelvis

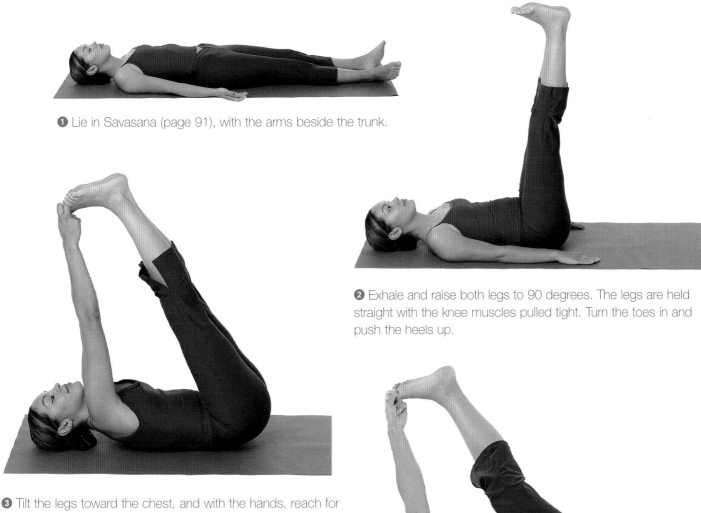

❶ Lie in Savasana (page 91), with the arms beside the trunk.

❷ Exhale and raise both legs to 90 degrees. The legs are held straight with the knee muscles pulled tight. Turn the toes in and push the heels up.

❸ Tilt the legs toward the chest, and with the hands, reach for the ankles or toes. Hold for a few seconds, breathing normally.

❹ Exhale and firmly clasp the toes to pull the legs as wide apart as is comfortable. Hold for 20–30 seconds. Release the hold on the feet and return the legs to the floor. Repeat once more.

setu bandhasana **bridge posture**

Setu means "bridge" and *bandha* means "formation." In Setu bandhasana, the legs, hips, and back are raised and the body resembles a bridge shape.

level: Beginner/Intermediate

benefits • Tones the legs and arms • Increases the flexibility of the spine • Strengthens the wrists and ankles

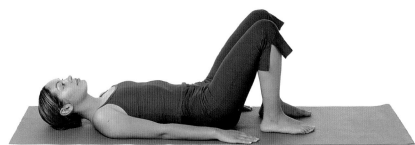

❶ Lie in Savasana (page 91), with the arms beside the trunk.

❷ Bend the knees, with the feet about a foot apart on the floor. Draw the soles of the feet toward the buttocks.

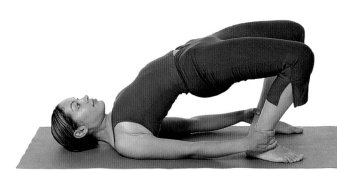

❸ With the hands firmly clasp the ankles. Inhale to raise the hips and the back off the floor. Arch the spine to elevate the hips further. Breathe evenly, holding for 20–30 seconds. Release the hold on the ankles and gently lower the hips and the back onto the floor.

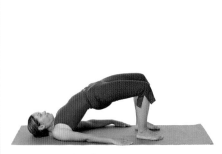

VARIATIONS: beginner
The arms are by the side of the body, with the palms facing down. The hips and back are raised as above.

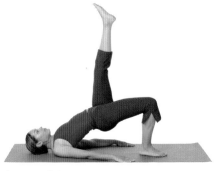

intermediate
The arms are by the side of the body, with the palms facing down. The hips and the back are raised as above. Exhale and raise the right leg up straight. Repeat, raising the left leg.

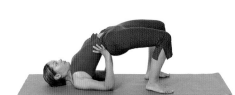

intermediate
Bend the arms, shifting the weight onto the upper arms and elbow. Place the palms under the upper back. The fingers are pointing outward.

matsyasana **fish posture**

Matsya means "fish." Matsyasana is the counterposture to Sarvangasana (page 117) and should ideally be practiced after it. The spine is arched and head tilted back to give a streamlined shape.

level: Beginner

caution: The front of the neck is strongly stretched. If this results in discomfort, avoid this stretch. Instead practice Paschimottanasana (page 87).

benefits • Regulates the function of the thyroid and parathyroid glands • Promotes deeper breathing • Releases neck and shoulder tension • Deters colds

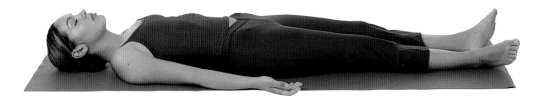

❶ Lie in Savasana (page 91), with the arms beside the trunk.

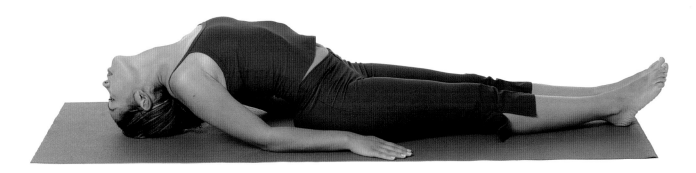

❷ Place the palms flat on the floor. Point the toes away from the body. Pressing down on the elbow, exhale to raise the chest up and tilt the head back. Arch the spine and compress the back of the neck to allow the crown of the head to rest on the floor. Breathe deeply, holding for 20–30 seconds. Inhale when returning to Savasana.

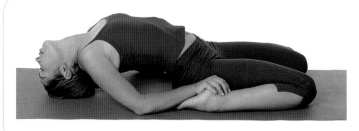

VARIATION: intermediate

From Vajrasana (page 51), lean back and rest on the elbows. Tilt the head back, sliding the elbows forward to enable the crown of the head to rest on the floor.

chakrasana **wheel posture**

Chakra means "energy center" or "wheel." Chakrasana requires considerable upper-body strength and a supple spine. In this strong stretch all the chakras are stimulated, energizing the mind and body.

level: Intermediate/Advanced

caution: This posture requires a strong and supple spine and should be attempted only by someone who has been practicing yoga for some time.

benefits • Stimulates the entire circulatory system • Strengthens the spine • Tones the legs, abdomen, and arms • Refreshes the body

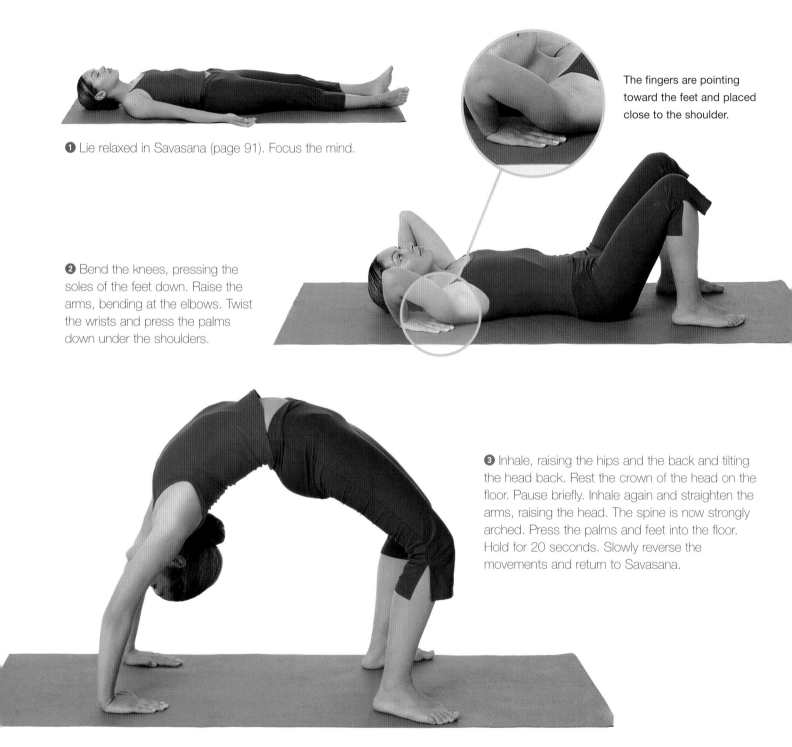

❶ Lie relaxed in Savasana (page 91). Focus the mind.

The fingers are pointing toward the feet and placed close to the shoulder.

❷ Bend the knees, pressing the soles of the feet down. Raise the arms, bending at the elbows. Twist the wrists and press the palms down under the shoulders.

❸ Inhale, raising the hips and the back and tilting the head back. Rest the crown of the head on the floor. Pause briefly. Inhale again and straighten the arms, raising the head. The spine is now strongly arched. Press the palms and feet into the floor. Hold for 20 seconds. Slowly reverse the movements and return to Savasana.

supta vrksasana lying-down tree posture

Supta means "lying down" and *vrksa* means "tree." Supta vrksasana prepares the feet, knees, and legs for adopting Padmasana (page 63).

level: Beginner

benefits • Increases the flexibility of the ankles, knees, and hips

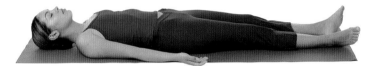

❶ Lie in Savasana (page 91), with the arms beside the trunk.

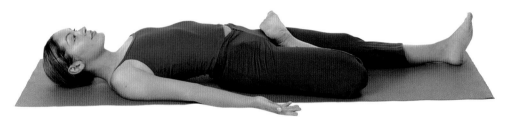

❷ Bend the right leg and place the foot either on the left thigh with the sole of the foot turned upward or against the inner left thigh. Keep the left leg firm with the toes pointing up.

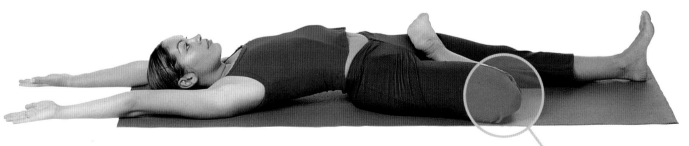

❸ Inhale and extend the arms over the head. The palms are facing up with the fingers stretched. Hold for 30–60 seconds, breathing deeply. Repeat on the other side.

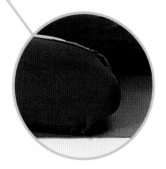

Press the knee downward.

Yoga is stilling the activities of the mind.

Patanjali's *Yoga Sutra*

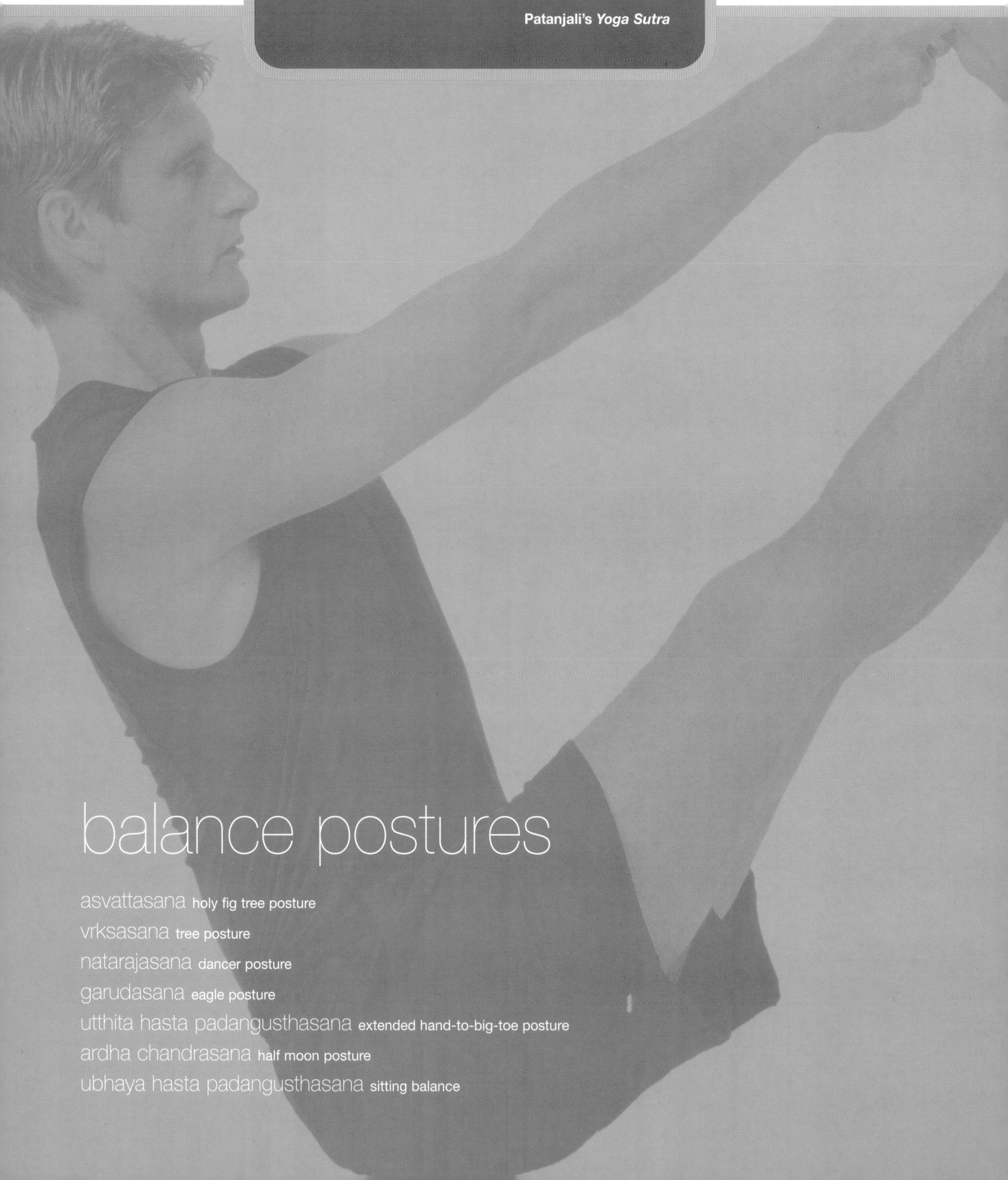

balance postures

asvattasana holy fig tree posture

vrksasana tree posture

natarajasana dancer posture

garudasana eagle posture

utthita hasta padangusthasana extended hand-to-big-toe posture

ardha chandrasana half moon posture

ubhaya hasta padangusthasana sitting balance

asvattasana holy fig tree posture

Asvatta means "sacred fig tree." The holy fig tree or Pipal (Bodhi) tree is a strong and robust tree. Unlike other trees, it releases oxygen at night. In Indian mythology, the Pipal tree is associated with the abode of the god Shiva. In Asvattasana, three limbs are raised and stretched in three different planes.

level: Beginner

benefits • Promotes deeper breathing • Improves energy • Improves circulation

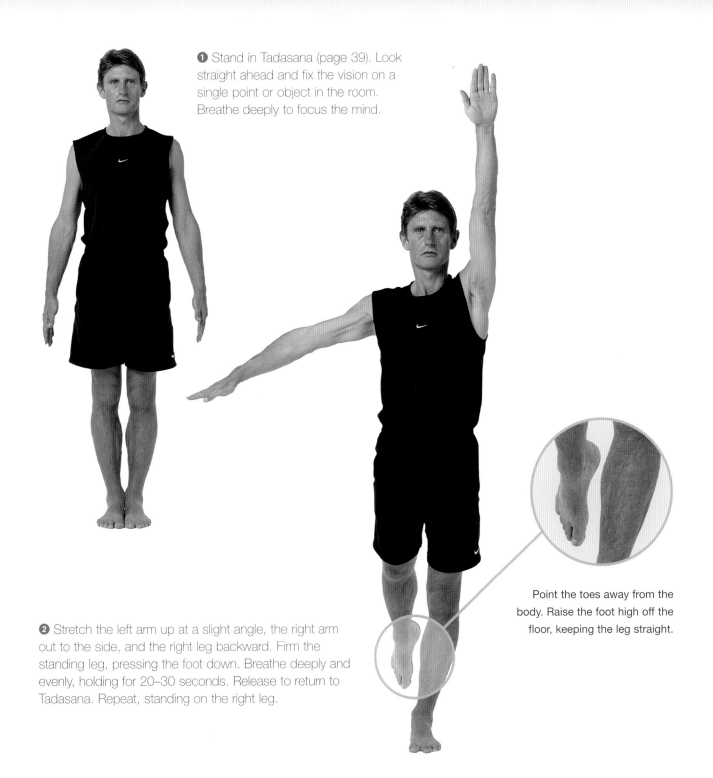

❶ Stand in Tadasana (page 39). Look straight ahead and fix the vision on a single point or object in the room. Breathe deeply to focus the mind.

❷ Stretch the left arm up at a slight angle, the right arm out to the side, and the right leg backward. Firm the standing leg, pressing the foot down. Breathe deeply and evenly, holding for 20–30 seconds. Release to return to Tadasana. Repeat, standing on the right leg.

Point the toes away from the body. Raise the foot high off the floor, keeping the leg straight.

vrksasana **tree posture**

Vrksa means "tree." Vrksasana is a graceful balance posture. The foot pressing into the ground is like the root of the tree and the arms stretch up like the branches of the tree. The position of the raised foot is akin to the Half-lotus foot position (page 63). The ancient yogis stayed in this posture for hours on end as a form of *tapas*, or austerity.

level: Beginner

practice: If balancing is difficult, stand against a wall to avoid falling. The raised foot can be placed at the side of the knee.

benefits • Develops memory and concentration • Improves poise and posture • Firms and tones the muscles of the legs, back, and chest

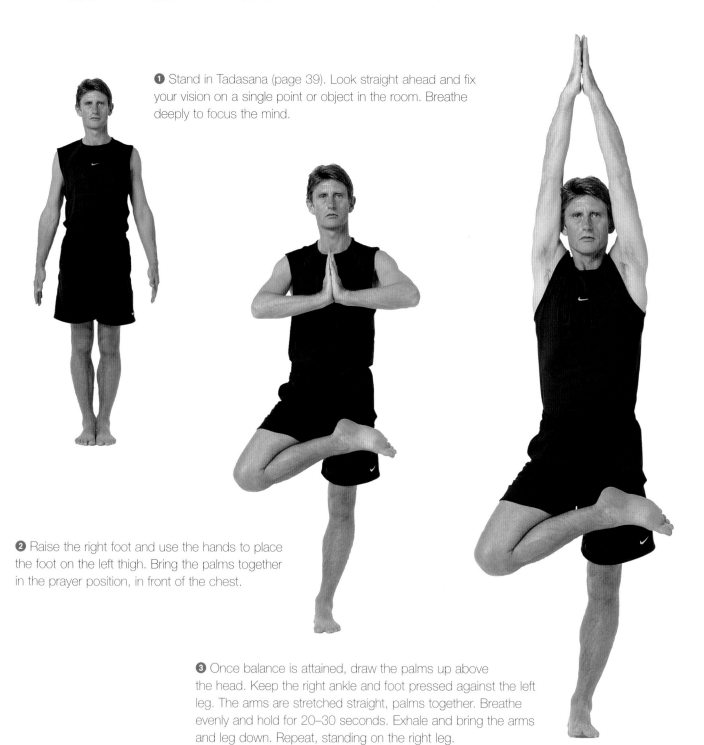

❶ Stand in Tadasana (page 39). Look straight ahead and fix your vision on a single point or object in the room. Breathe deeply to focus the mind.

❷ Raise the right foot and use the hands to place the foot on the left thigh. Bring the palms together in the prayer position, in front of the chest.

❸ Once balance is attained, draw the palms up above the head. Keep the right ankle and foot pressed against the left leg. The arms are stretched straight, palms together. Breathe evenly and hold for 20–30 seconds. Exhale and bring the arms and leg down. Repeat, standing on the right leg.

natarajasana dancer posture

Nataraj means "Lord of the Dance." Natarajasana is based on the cosmic dance, which Lord Shiva performs at the beginning and end of each cycle of creation. Lord Shiva is regarded as the source of the entire yoga system. The image of Shiva Nataraj dancing in a ring of fire is frequently seen in Hindu sculpture.

level: Beginner

benefits • Tones the nervous system • Improves physical and mental poise • Strengthens the legs and spine

Firmly clasp fingers on the foot to raise the foot as high as possible.

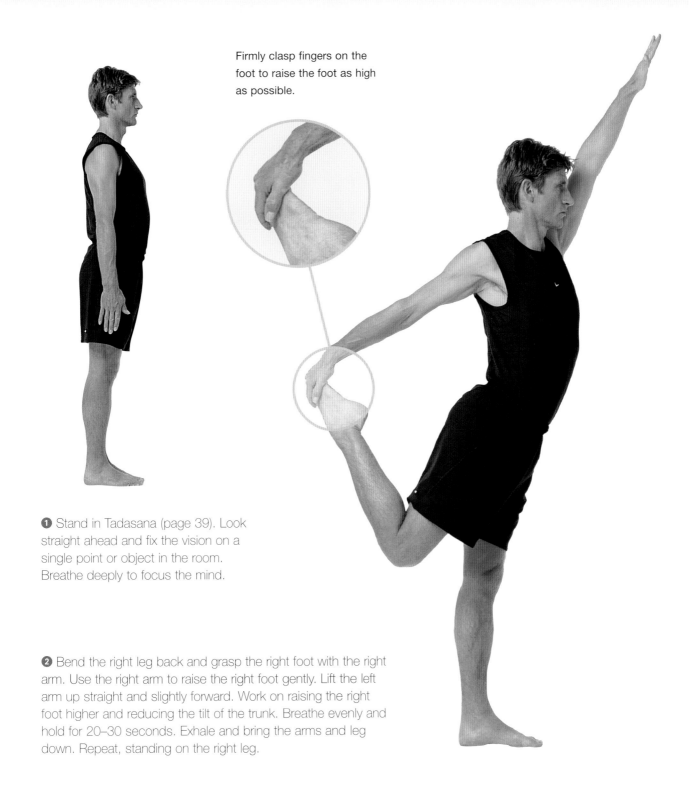

❶ Stand in Tadasana (page 39). Look straight ahead and fix the vision on a single point or object in the room. Breathe deeply to focus the mind.

❷ Bend the right leg back and grasp the right foot with the right arm. Use the right arm to raise the right foot gently. Lift the left arm up straight and slightly forward. Work on raising the right foot higher and reducing the tilt of the trunk. Breathe evenly and hold for 20–30 seconds. Exhale and bring the arms and leg down. Repeat, standing on the right leg.

garudasana **eagle posture**

Garuda in Hindi mythology is the eagle deity, represented as having the beak and wings of an eagle and the body of a man. Garudasana requires a great deal of suppleness in the legs and shoulders.

level: Intermediate/Advanced

benefits • Improves the concentration • Improves circulation to the extremities • Strengthens the knees and ankles

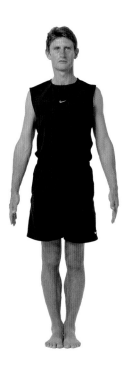

❶ Stand in Tadasana (page 39). Look straight ahead and fix the vision on a single point or object in the room. Breathe deeply to focus the mind.

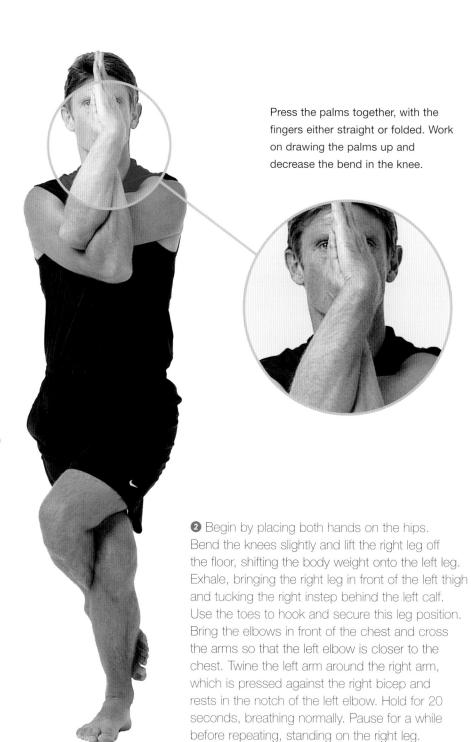

Press the palms together, with the fingers either straight or folded. Work on drawing the palms up and decrease the bend in the knee.

❷ Begin by placing both hands on the hips. Bend the knees slightly and lift the right leg off the floor, shifting the body weight onto the left leg. Exhale, bringing the right leg in front of the left thigh and tucking the right instep behind the left calf. Use the toes to hook and secure this leg position. Bring the elbows in front of the chest and cross the arms so that the left elbow is closer to the chest. Twine the left arm around the right arm, which is pressed against the right bicep and rests in the notch of the left elbow. Hold for 20 seconds, breathing normally. Pause for a while before repeating, standing on the right leg.

uttihita hasta padangusthasana **extended hand-to-big-toe**

Uttihita means "extended," *hasta* means "hand," and *padangustha* means "big toe." Uttihita hasta padangusthasana gives a powerful stretch to the raised leg combined with graceful balance.

level: Intermediate

practice: If balancing is difficult, place the foot on a table and use a belt to link foot and hand.

benefits • Strengthens the legs and lower back • Increases physical and mental poise • Limbers up the hips

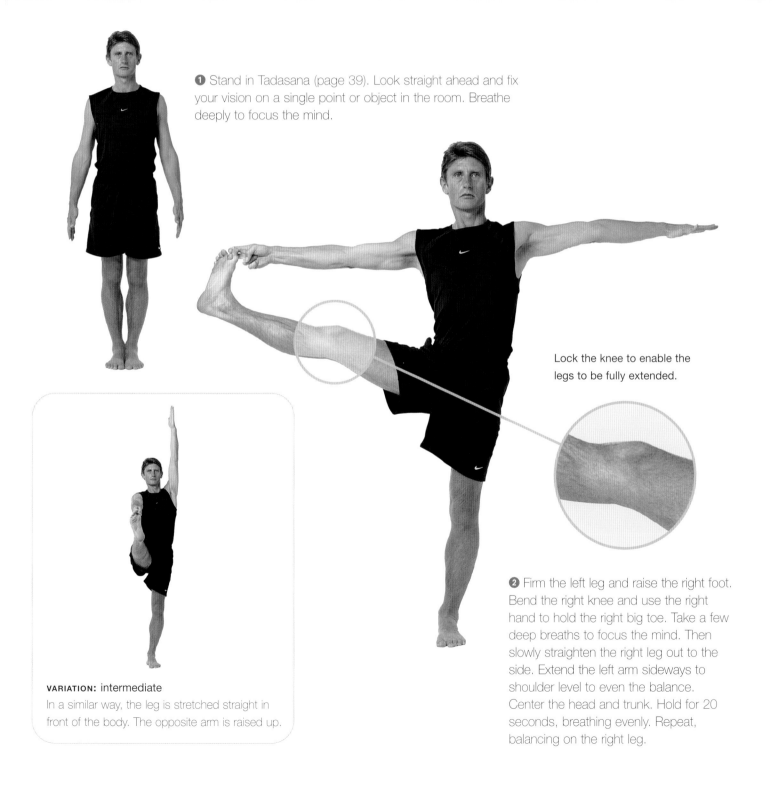

❶ Stand in Tadasana (page 39). Look straight ahead and fix your vision on a single point or object in the room. Breathe deeply to focus the mind.

Lock the knee to enable the legs to be fully extended.

VARIATION: intermediate
In a similar way, the leg is stretched straight in front of the body. The opposite arm is raised up.

❷ Firm the left leg and raise the right foot. Bend the right knee and use the right hand to hold the right big toe. Take a few deep breaths to focus the mind. Then slowly straighten the right leg out to the side. Extend the left arm sideways to shoulder level to even the balance. Center the head and trunk. Hold for 20 seconds, breathing evenly. Repeat, balancing on the right leg.

ardha chandrasana   half moon posture

Ardha means "half" and *chandra* means "moon." Ardha chandrasana is a lateral balance posture with the trunk tipped sideways. All limbs are stretched in three planes.

level: Intermediate/Advanced

practice: Place the lower hand on a block, if necessary.

benefits • Regulates the digestive system • Improves poise • Strengthens the ankles and legs

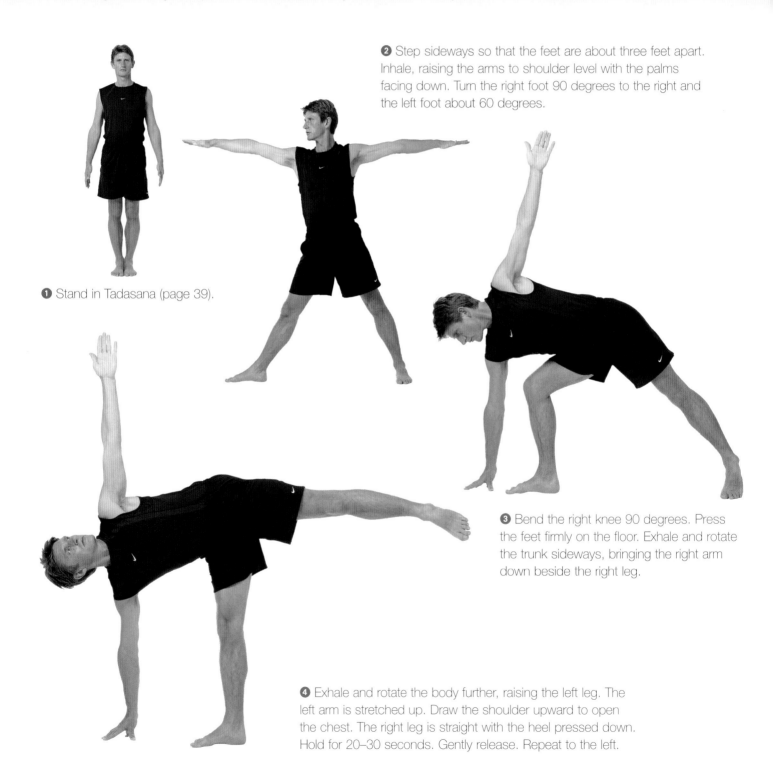

❶ Stand in Tadasana (page 39).

❷ Step sideways so that the feet are about three feet apart. Inhale, raising the arms to shoulder level with the palms facing down. Turn the right foot 90 degrees to the right and the left foot about 60 degrees.

❸ Bend the right knee 90 degrees. Press the feet firmly on the floor. Exhale and rotate the trunk sideways, bringing the right arm down beside the right leg.

❹ Exhale and rotate the body further, raising the left leg. The left arm is stretched up. Draw the shoulder upward to open the chest. The right leg is straight with the heel pressed down. Hold for 20–30 seconds. Gently release. Repeat to the left.

ubhaya hasta padangusthasana **sitting balance**

Ubhaya means "both," *hasta* means "hand," and *padangustha* means "big toe." Ubhaya hasta padangusthasana involves balancing on the buttocks with the back and legs kept straight.

level: Intermediate

practice: Initially hold the ankles rather than the toes. If there is a tendency to topple backward, place cushions behind to give support.

benefits • Strengthens and tones the arms, legs, and abdomen • Limbers up the hips • Improves the circulation • Improves the digestive system

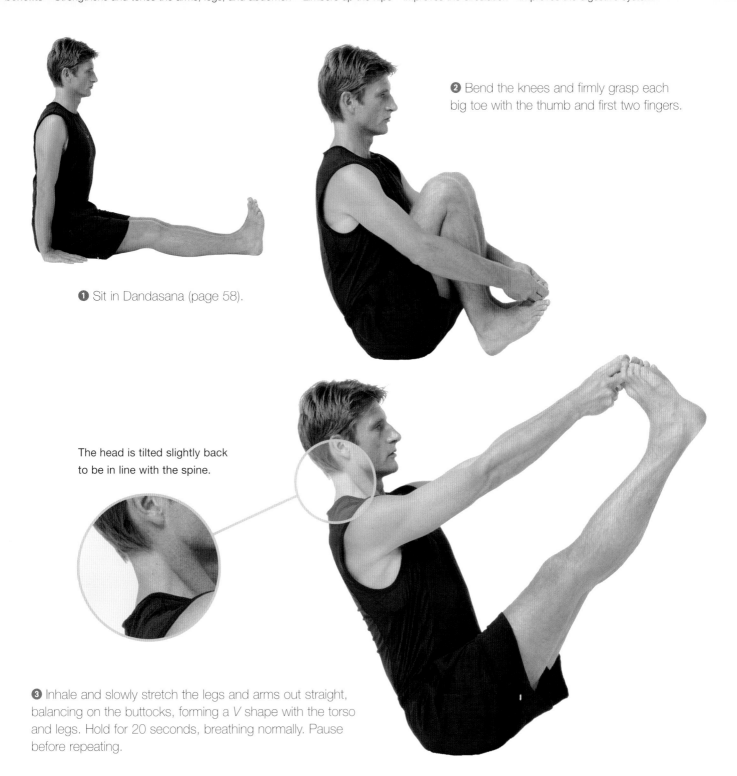

❷ Bend the knees and firmly grasp each big toe with the thumb and first two fingers.

❶ Sit in Dandasana (page 58).

The head is tilted slightly back to be in line with the spine.

❸ Inhale and slowly stretch the legs and arms out straight, balancing on the buttocks, forming a *V* shape with the torso and legs. Hold for 20 seconds, breathing normally. Pause before repeating.

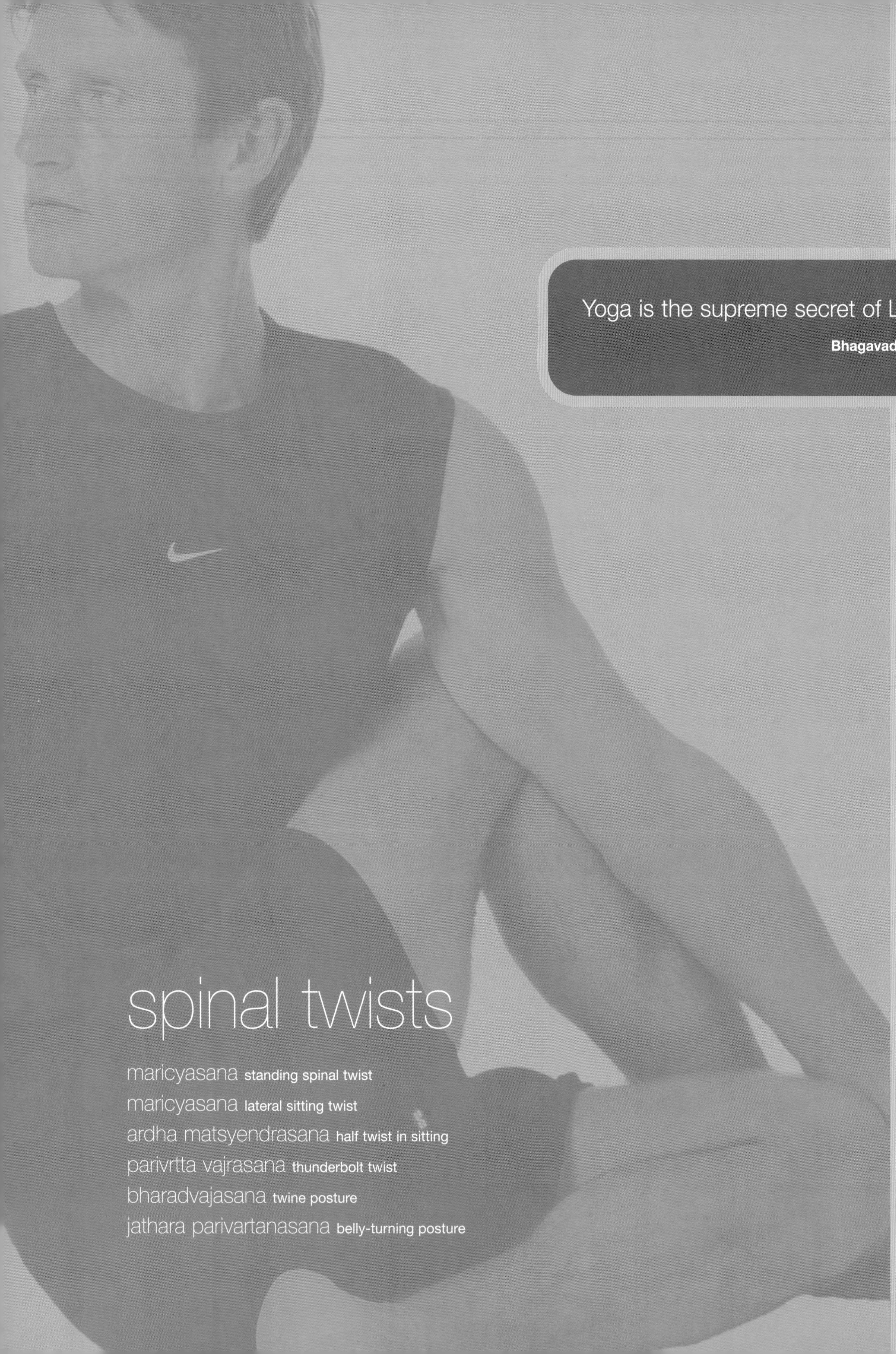

Yoga is the supreme secret of Life.

Bhagavad Gita

spinal twists

maricyasana standing spinal twist

maricyasana lateral sitting twist

ardha matsyendrasana half twist in sitting

parivrtta vajrasana thunderbolt twist

bharadvajasana twine posture

jathara parivartanasana belly-turning posture

maricyasana **standing spinal twist**

Marici is the name of a sage. In Maricyasana, the spine is given a gentle twist. By rotating the trunk 90 degrees, the back muscles are stretched and invigorated.

level: Beginner

benefits • Relieves back pain • Improves the function of the digestive system • Increases the flexibility of the hips and spine

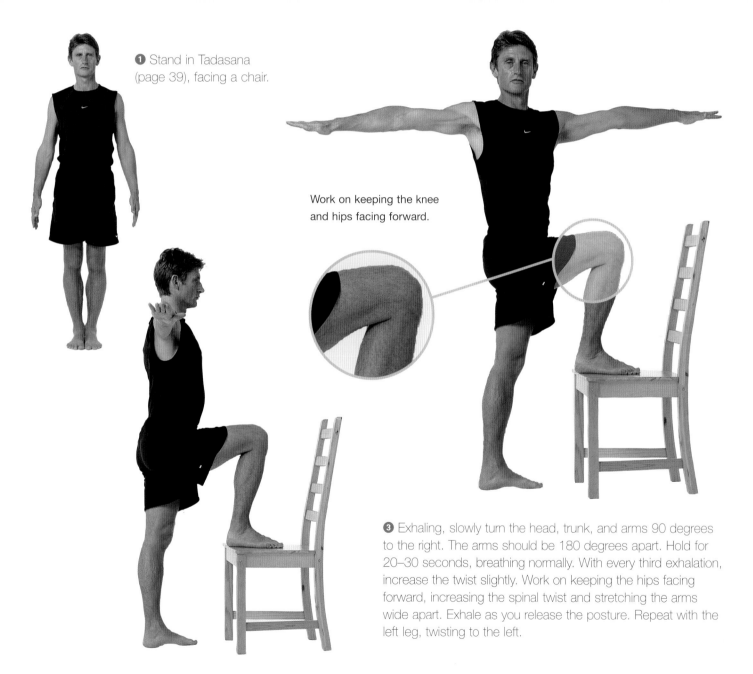

❶ Stand in Tadasana (page 39), facing a chair.

Work on keeping the knee and hips facing forward.

❸ Exhaling, slowly turn the head, trunk, and arms 90 degrees to the right. The arms should be 180 degrees apart. Hold for 20–30 seconds, breathing normally. With every third exhalation, increase the twist slightly. Work on keeping the hips facing forward, increasing the spinal twist and stretching the arms wide apart. Exhale as you release the posture. Repeat with the left leg, twisting to the left.

❷ Position the right foot on the seat of the chair. Inhale and raise the arms to shoulder level, with the palms turned down. The toes and heels should face forward. Firm the legs and press the feet down.

maricyasana **lateral sitting twist**

In this variation of Maricyasana, the spine is twisted gently from a sitting position.

level: Beginner

benefits • Relieves back pain • Improves the function of the digestive system • Tones the liver, spleen, and pancreas

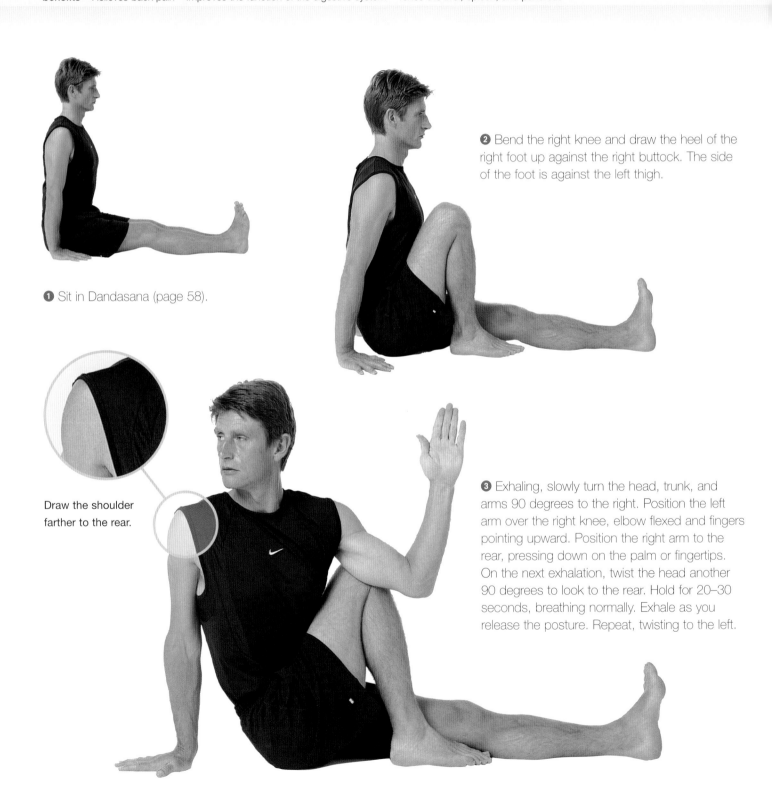

❶ Sit in Dandasana (page 58).

❷ Bend the right knee and draw the heel of the right foot up against the right buttock. The side of the foot is against the left thigh.

Draw the shoulder farther to the rear.

❸ Exhaling, slowly turn the head, trunk, and arms 90 degrees to the right. Position the left arm over the right knee, elbow flexed and fingers pointing upward. Position the right arm to the rear, pressing down on the palm or fingertips. On the next exhalation, twist the head another 90 degrees to look to the rear. Hold for 20–30 seconds, breathing normally. Exhale as you release the posture. Repeat, twisting to the left.

ardha matsyendrasana **half twist in sitting**

Ardha means "half" and Matsyendra is the "Lord of Fishes," who is considered to be the first teacher of yoga. In Ardha matsyendrasana, particular attention needs to be paid to the position of the lower limbs to give a strong twist to the spine.

level: Intermediate

benefits • Lubricates the spine and hip joints • Cleanses the liver • Relieves constipation • Brings harmony to the body

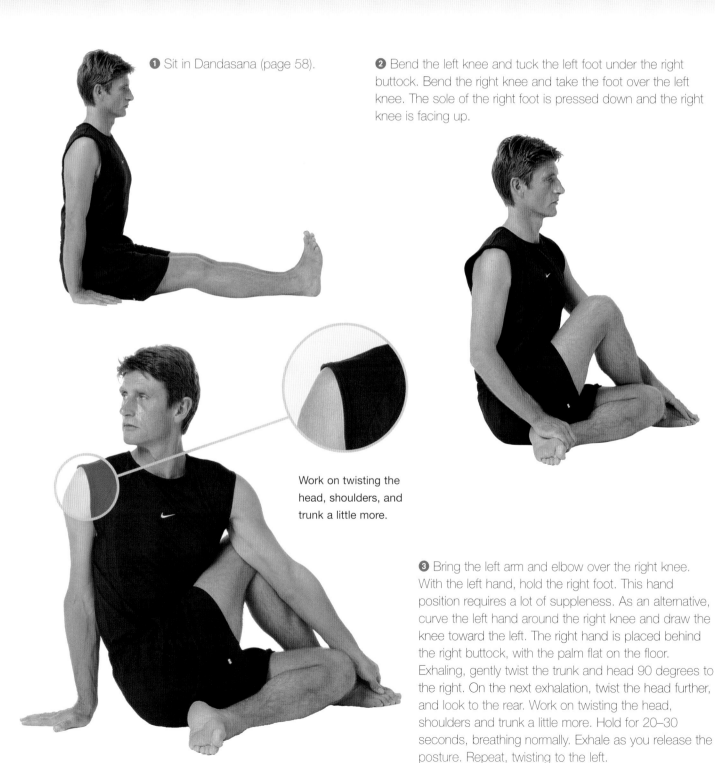

❶ Sit in Dandasana (page 58).

❷ Bend the left knee and tuck the left foot under the right buttock. Bend the right knee and take the foot over the left knee. The sole of the right foot is pressed down and the right knee is facing up.

Work on twisting the head, shoulders, and trunk a little more.

❸ Bring the left arm and elbow over the right knee. With the left hand, hold the right foot. This hand position requires a lot of suppleness. As an alternative, curve the left hand around the right knee and draw the knee toward the left. The right hand is placed behind the right buttock, with the palm flat on the floor. Exhaling, gently twist the trunk and head 90 degrees to the right. On the next exhalation, twist the head further, and look to the rear. Work on twisting the head, shoulders and trunk a little more. Hold for 20–30 seconds, breathing normally. Exhale as you release the posture. Repeat, twisting to the left.

parivrtta vajrasana **thunderbolt twist**

Parivrtta means "reverse" or "rotated" and *vajra* means "thunderbolt." Parivrtta vajrasana is one of the simplest spinal twists, carried out in a sitting position, and it provides a gentle massaging twist to the lumbar regions.

level: Beginner

benefits • Soothes lower back pain • Massages the abdominal organs

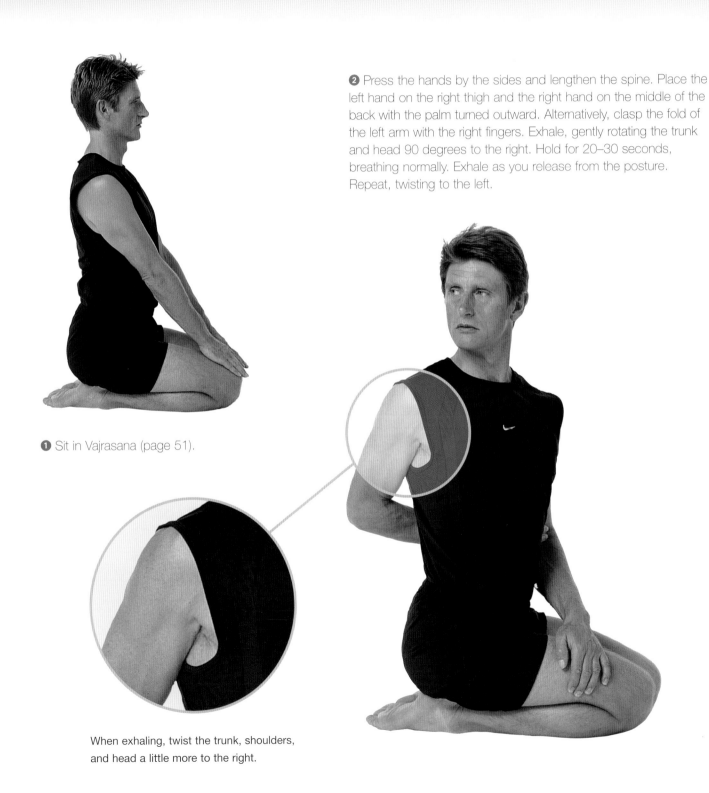

2 Press the hands by the sides and lengthen the spine. Place the left hand on the right thigh and the right hand on the middle of the back with the palm turned outward. Alternatively, clasp the fold of the left arm with the right fingers. Exhale, gently rotating the trunk and head 90 degrees to the right. Hold for 20–30 seconds, breathing normally. Exhale as you release from the posture. Repeat, twisting to the left.

1 Sit in Vajrasana (page 51).

When exhaling, twist the trunk, shoulders, and head a little more to the right.

bharadvajasana **twine posture**

Bharadvaja is the name of a sage. Bharadvajasana is a simple sitting twist, which benefits the dorsal and lumbar regions. The legs are displaced and folded to the side, enabling the twist to begin at the base of the spine and work up to the neck. This posture can be carried out even if the back is very stiff.

level: Beginner

benefits • Relieves stiffness in the neck, shoulders, and lower back

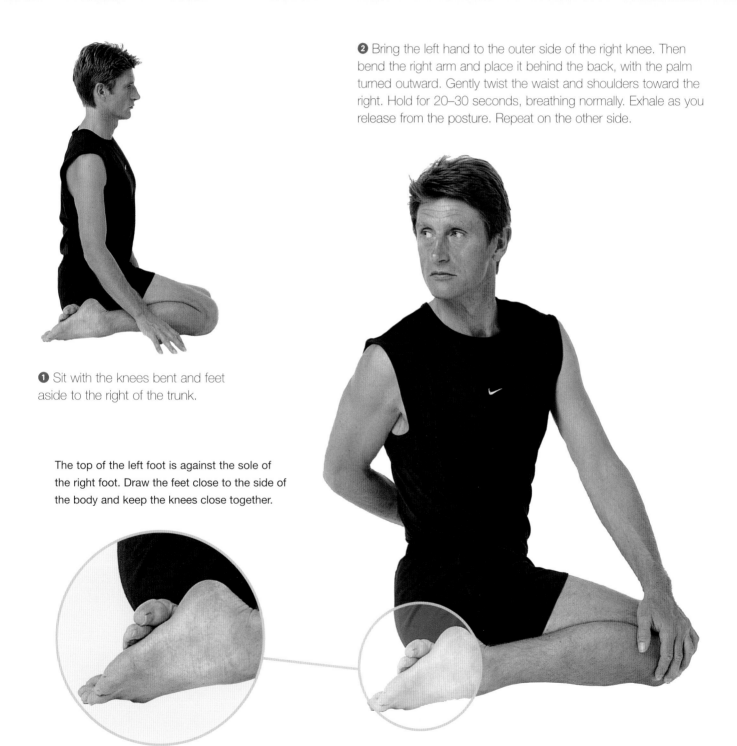

❷ Bring the left hand to the outer side of the right knee. Then bend the right arm and place it behind the back, with the palm turned outward. Gently twist the waist and shoulders toward the right. Hold for 20–30 seconds, breathing normally. Exhale as you release from the posture. Repeat on the other side.

❶ Sit with the knees bent and feet aside to the right of the trunk.

The top of the left foot is against the sole of the right foot. Draw the feet close to the side of the body and keep the knees close together.

jathara parivartanasana belly-turning posture

Jathara means "belly" or "stomach" and *parivartana* means "turning around." This posture involves twisting at the hips and abdomen. The weight of the legs, positioned sideways, stretches the lower back muscles and abdomen.

level: Beginner/Intermediate

benefits • Increases the flexibility of the spine and hips • Massages the internal organs of the abdomen

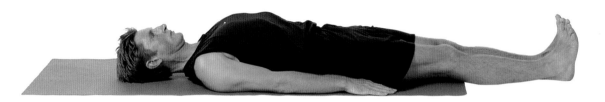

❶ Lie on your back, arms by your side, palms down, legs together and stretched out with toes pointing upward.

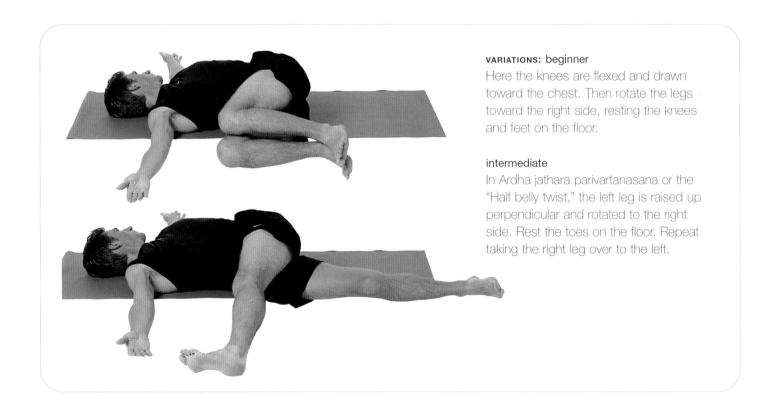

VARIATIONS: beginner
Here the knees are flexed and drawn toward the chest. Then rotate the legs toward the right side, resting the knees and feet on the floor.

intermediate
In Ardha jathara parivartanasana or the "Half belly twist," the left leg is raised up perpendicular and rotated to the right side. Rest the toes on the floor. Repeat taking the right leg over to the left.

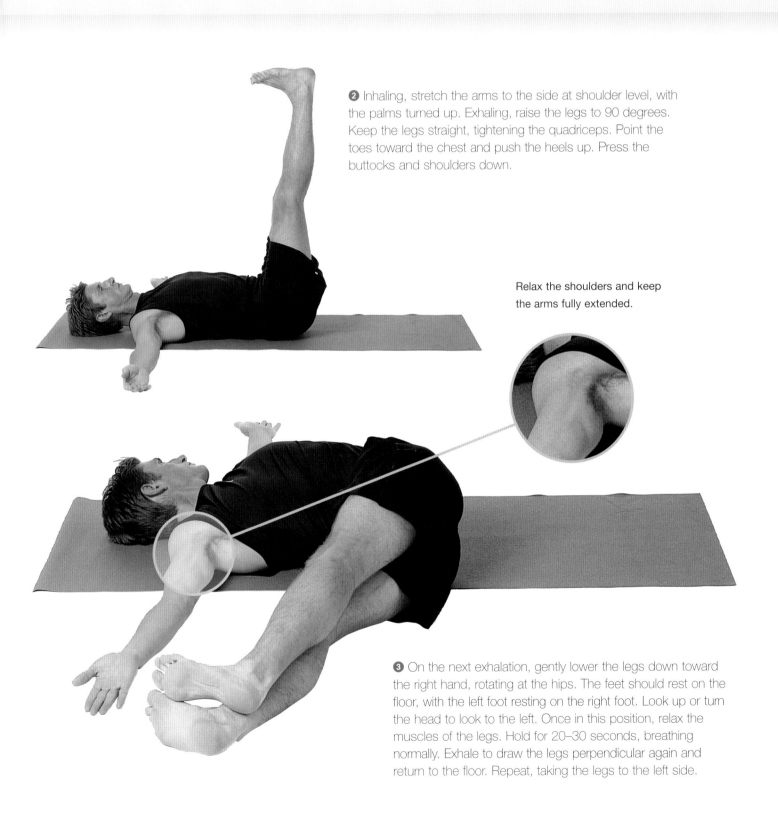

② Inhaling, stretch the arms to the side at shoulder level, with the palms turned up. Exhaling, raise the legs to 90 degrees. Keep the legs straight, tightening the quadriceps. Point the toes toward the chest and push the heels up. Press the buttocks and shoulders down.

Relax the shoulders and keep the arms fully extended.

③ On the next exhalation, gently lower the legs down toward the right hand, rotating at the hips. The feet should rest on the floor, with the left foot resting on the right foot. Look up or turn the head to look to the left. Once in this position, relax the muscles of the legs. Hold for 20–30 seconds, breathing normally. Exhale to draw the legs perpendicular again and return to the floor. Repeat, taking the legs to the left side.

Evenness (samatva) is called Yoga.

Bhagavad Gita

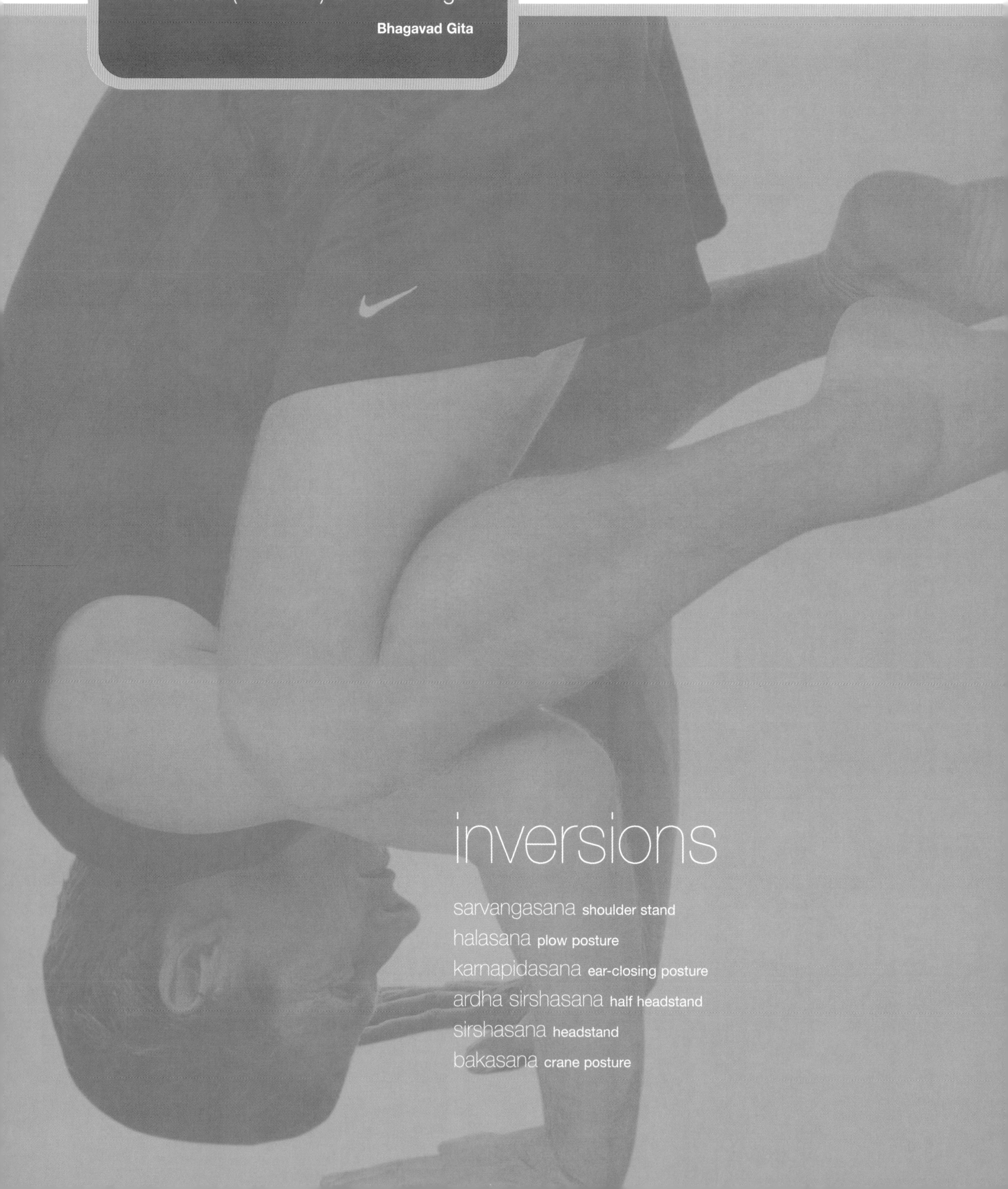

inversions

sarvangasana shoulder stand

halasana plow posture

karnapidasana ear-closing posture

ardha sirshasana half headstand

sirshasana headstand

bakasana crane posture

sarvangasana **shoulder stand**

Sarva means "all" or "complete," and *anga* means "body." Traditionally viewed as the "Queen of Postures," Sarvangasana is beneficial to the whole body. The flow of blood is reversed, increasing the blood supply to the face and brain and increasing the metabolic rate. A good counterposture is Matsyasana (page 97).

level: Intermediate

caution: Avoid if prone to high blood pressure, nasal problems, thyroid irregularities, or weak neck muscles, and during menstruation.

benefits • Tones the facial skin and prevents wrinkles • Firms the legs, abdomen, and arms • Regulates the function of the thyroid and parathyroid glands

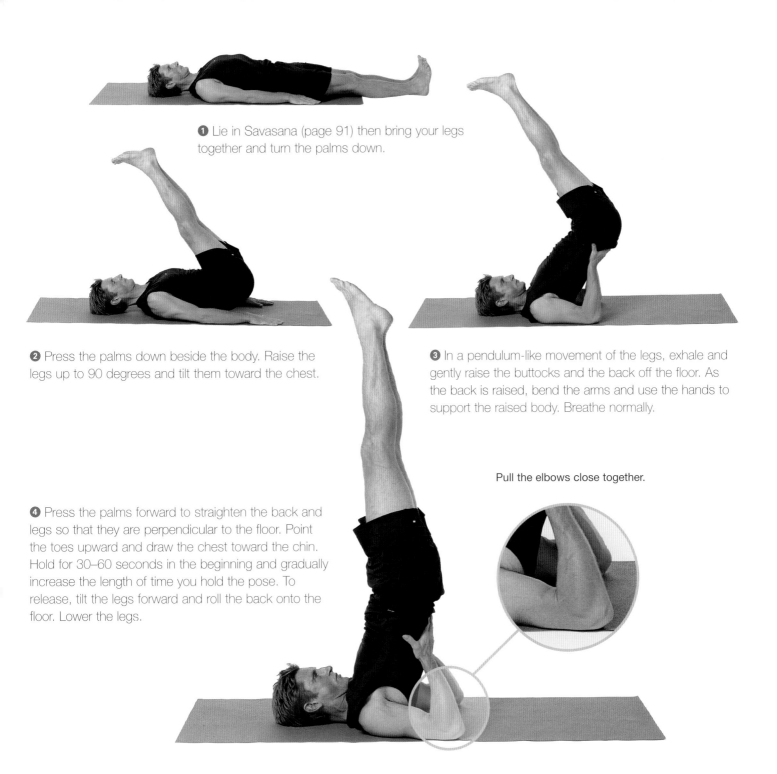

❶ Lie in Savasana (page 91) then bring your legs together and turn the palms down.

❷ Press the palms down beside the body. Raise the legs up to 90 degrees and tilt them toward the chest.

❸ In a pendulum-like movement of the legs, exhale and gently raise the buttocks and the back off the floor. As the back is raised, bend the arms and use the hands to support the raised body. Breathe normally.

Pull the elbows close together.

❹ Press the palms forward to straighten the back and legs so that they are perpendicular to the floor. Point the toes upward and draw the chest toward the chin. Hold for 30–60 seconds in the beginning and gradually increase the length of time you hold the pose. To release, tilt the legs forward and roll the back onto the floor. Lower the legs.

halasana **plow posture**

Hala means "plow." In Halasana, the body assumes the shape of an Indian plow. Halasana is often followed on from Sarvangasana (page 117).

level: Beginner/Intermediate

caution: If there is any discomfort or pain when holding in the posture, then avoid this posture. Women should avoid inversions during the menstrual period.

benefits • Expands the chest and cleanses the lungs, preventing chest ailments • Purifies the blood and cleanses the liver • Improves the flow of energy

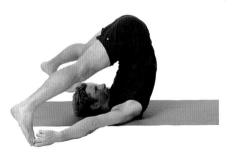

❶ Lie in Savasana (page 91). Then bring your legs together and turn the palms down.

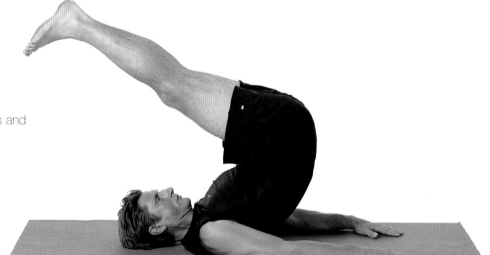

❷ Exhale to raise the legs 90 degrees and bring them over the chest and face.

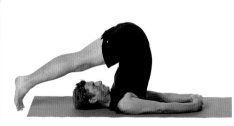

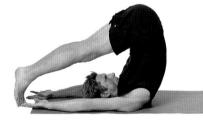

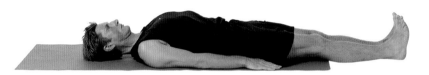

VARIATIONS: intermediate

Here the fingers are interlocked, with the palms facing the back.

Stretch the arms over the head, resting on the floor with the fingers pointing toward the toes.

From the previous position, take the feet wide apart and let the arms follow the span of the legs.

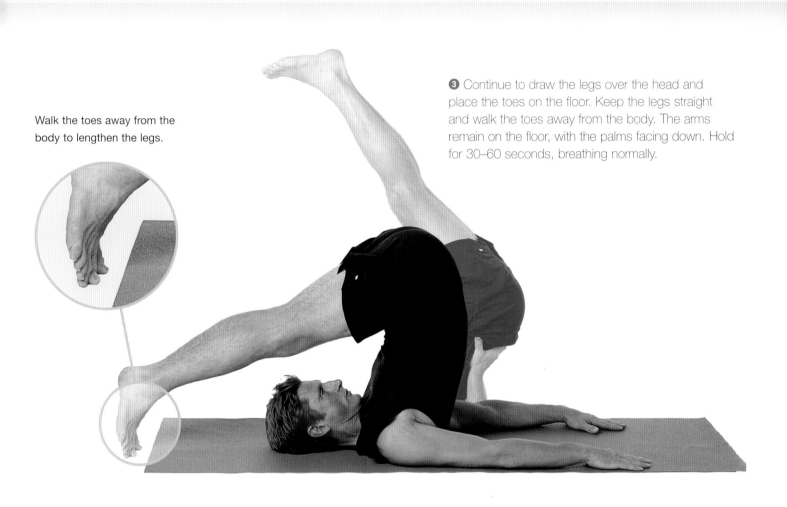

Walk the toes away from the
body to lengthen the legs.

❸ Continue to draw the legs over the head and
place the toes on the floor. Keep the legs straight
and walk the toes away from the body. The arms
remain on the floor, with the palms facing down. Hold
for 30–60 seconds, breathing normally.

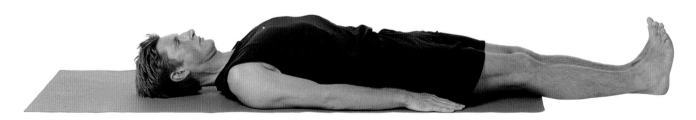

❹ Exhale to gently stretch the legs back onto the floor.

karnapidasana ear-closing posture

Karna means "ears" and *pida* means "pressure." This posture can be followed on from Halasana (pages 118–119). In this posture, the senses are momentarily withdrawn from the surroundings. The mind is rested and calmed.

level: Beginner/Intermediate

caution: Women should avoid inversions during the menstrual period.

benefits • Rejuvenates the mind and body

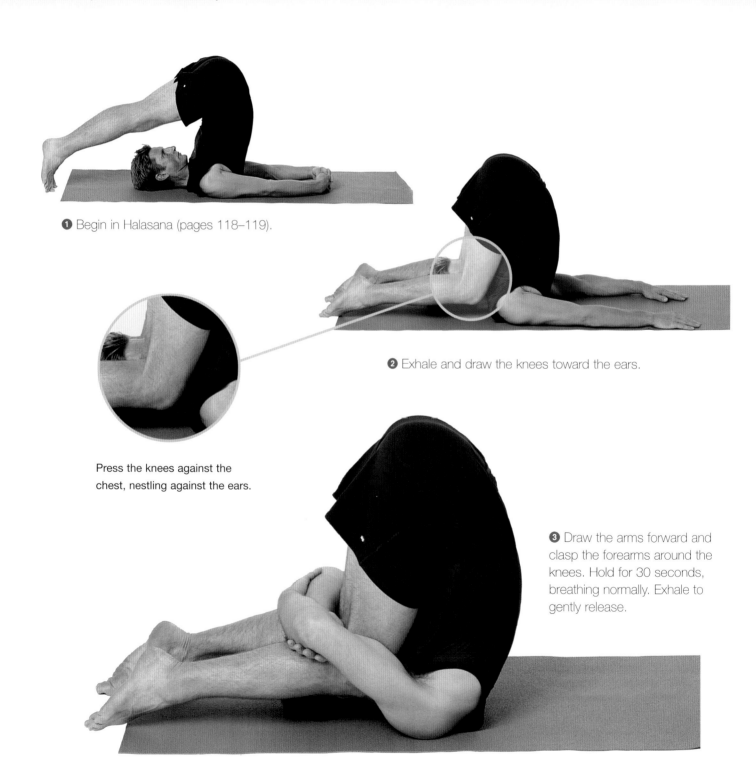

❶ Begin in Halasana (pages 118–119).

❷ Exhale and draw the knees toward the ears.

Press the knees against the chest, nestling against the ears.

❸ Draw the arms forward and clasp the forearms around the knees. Hold for 30 seconds, breathing normally. Exhale to gently release.

ardha sirshasana **half headstand**

Ardha means "half" and *sirsha* means "head." In this posture the body is partially inverted. To develop the skill to perform Sirshasana (page 122), practice Sarvangasana (page 117) and Ardha sirshasana regularly.

level: Intermediate

caution: Women should avoid inversions during the menstrual period.

benefits • Tones the legs and arms • Strengthens the spine • Improves the memory

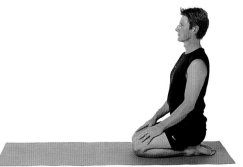
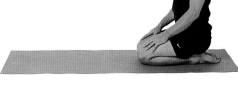

❶ Sit in Vajrasana (page 51). Breathe evenly and focus the mind.

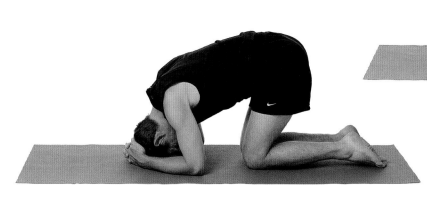

❷ Bend forward and rest the elbows and forearms on the floor in front.

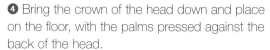

❸ Keep the elbows pressed down and move the hands forward so that the fingers can be interlocked. Make a tripod shape with the palms and forearms.

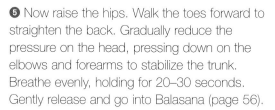

❹ Bring the crown of the head down and place on the floor, with the palms pressed against the back of the head.

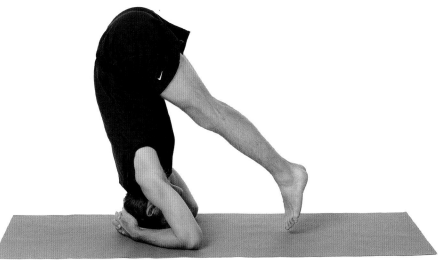

❺ Now raise the hips. Walk the toes forward to straighten the back. Gradually reduce the pressure on the head, pressing down on the elbows and forearms to stabilize the trunk. Breathe evenly, holding for 20–30 seconds. Gently release and go into Balasana (page 56).

sirshasana **headstand**

Sirsha means "head." In Sirshasana the entire body is inverted. The heart is able to rest briefly, as the flow of blood is reversed. Traditionally viewed as the "King of Postures," Sirshasana has immense benefits to the entire body. Mastery of Sarvangasana (page 117) is necessary before Sirshasana is attempted. Practice this posture against a wall.

level: Advanced

caution: If you have high blood pressure or weak eyes, you should avoid this stretch. Avoid inversions during the menstrual period.

benefits • Tones the legs, abdomen, and arms • Invigorates the brain and improves the memory • Nourishes the heart • Develops poise and agility

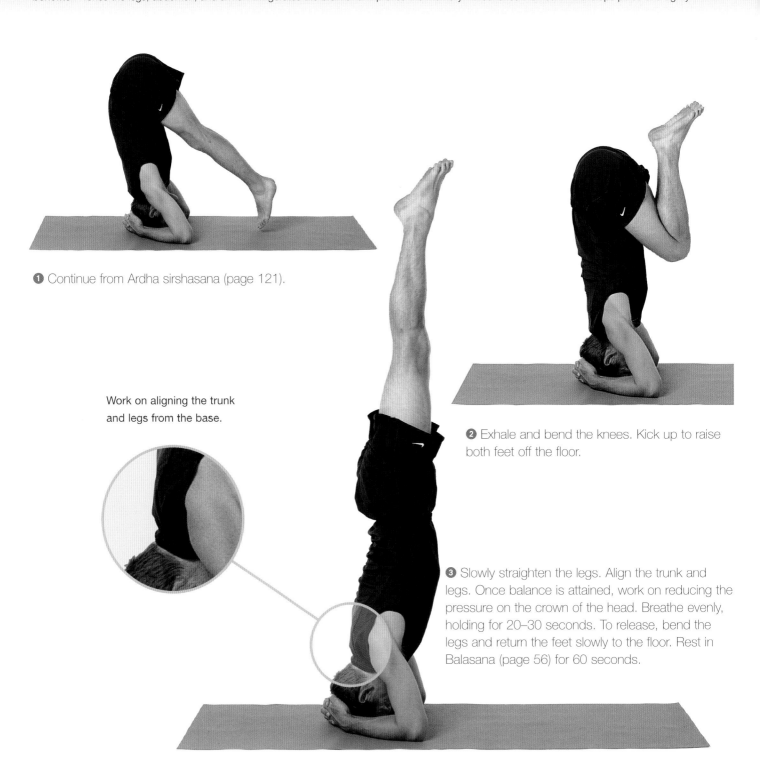

❶ Continue from Ardha sirshasana (page 121).

Work on aligning the trunk and legs from the base.

❷ Exhale and bend the knees. Kick up to raise both feet off the floor.

❸ Slowly straighten the legs. Align the trunk and legs. Once balance is attained, work on reducing the pressure on the crown of the head. Breathe evenly, holding for 20–30 seconds. To release, bend the legs and return the feet slowly to the floor. Rest in Balasana (page 56) for 60 seconds.

bakasana crane posture

Baka means "crane." This posture is based on the crane, which is a tall, wading bird with a long, elegant neck, long legs, and a straight beak. It treads in still water, with head bent down, looking for fish. At first the posture appears awkward to accomplish, but with practice can be mastered and enjoyed.

level: Intermediate

caution: Avoid inversions during the menstrual period.

benefits • Strengthens the shoulders, arms, wrists, and back • Improves the circulation

❶ Sit in Vajrasana (page 51).

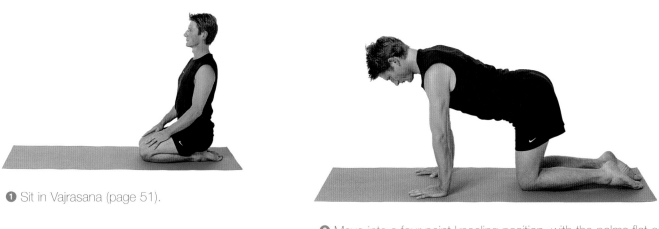

❷ Move into a four-point kneeling position, with the palms flat on the floor and the toes turned out.

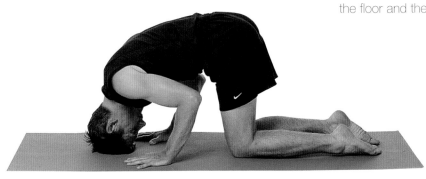

❸ Bring the crown of the head to rest on the floor. The head is placed about four inches in front of the hands. The elbows are raised and bent to 90 degrees. Turn the toes in.

Press the shins against the upper arms to give stability.

❹ Lift the right knee onto the right elbow and the left knee onto the left elbow, raising the feet off the floor as the weight of the legs is transferred to the elbows. Hold for 20–30 seconds, and gently release. A three-point headstand can be carried out from Bakasana by straightening the legs.

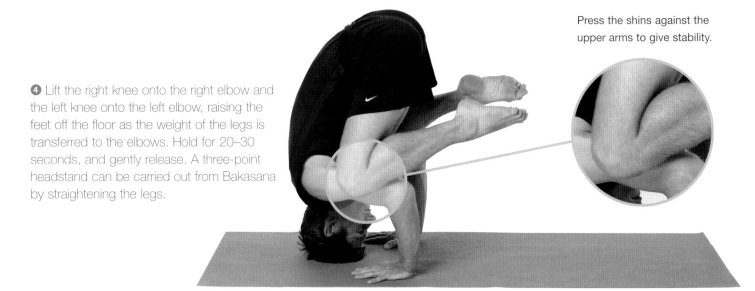

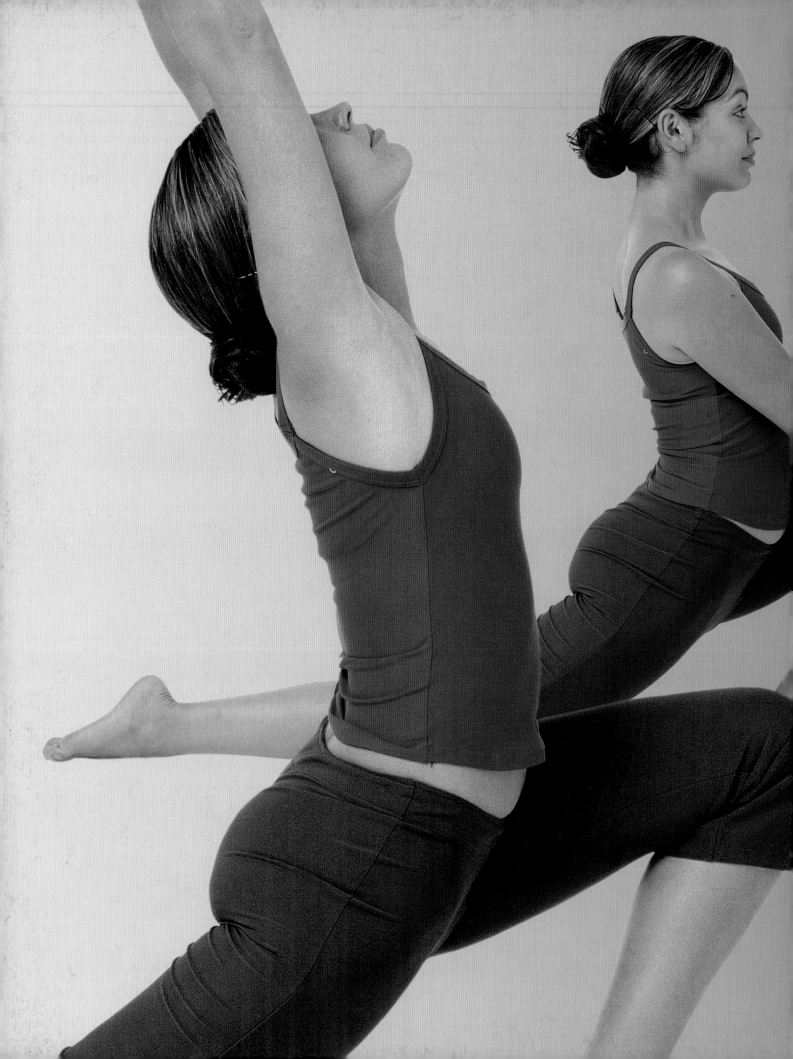

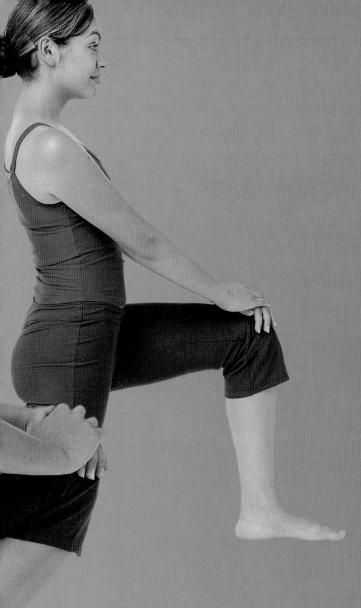

part 3

progressive yoga program

for home practice

This is a progressive program of four sessions graded at the beginner level. The program contains a variety of postures that will tone up different parts of the body. Each session can last either twenty, thirty, or forty minutes. The postures to be included in each time frame are marked out in Table 1. Each session can be repeated several times, until the postures are carried out with ease. With practice, as familiarity with the postures increases, the session plan can be adapted to suit your individual needs. When a posture is difficult or unsuitable to perform, then replace that posture with a more suitable one from the same section. When replacing a posture in the program, remember to incorporate a suitable counterstretch. When this program can be performed with relative ease, then move on to the intermediate program.

personal checklist

- Wear loose and comfortable clothes.

- Wait to practice yoga for at least two hours after a heavy meal.

- Warm-up exercises (pages 34–37) are important to prepare the muscles.

- Don't rush the postures—enjoy and explore each posture.

- Focus the mind and steady the breath when preparing to enter a posture.

- Unless stipulated, breathing should be carried through the nostrils.

- Use the relaxation poses between the postures: Balasana (page 56) and Savasana (page 91).

- Seek medical advice if pain or discomfort is experienced when practicing yoga.

- Be patient—regular practice is important to accrue the immense benefits of yoga.

table 1 beginner-level yoga program

session 1	20	30	40	session 2	20	30	40	session 3	20	30	40	session 4	20	30	40
warm-up exercises	•	•	•	warm-up exercises	•	•	•	warm-up exercises	•	•	•	warm-up exercises	•	•	•
urdhva hastottasana / upstretched arms posture	•	•	•	hanumanasana / hanuman posture	•	•	•	uttihita trikonasana / extended triangle	•	•	•	virabhadrasana / warrior posture	•	•	•
ardha uttanasana / half forward bend	•	•	•	utkatasana / squatting posture	•	•	•	ardha uttanasana / half forward bend	•	•	•	uttanasana / standing forward bend	•	•	•
nagasana / raised serpent	•	•	•	parighasana / cross-bar posture			•	vrksasana / tree posture			•	utkatasana / squatting posture			•
balasana / child's posture	•	•	•	balasana / child's posture	•	•	•	balasana / child's posture	•	•	•	balasana / child's posture	•	•	•
udhitta padasana / raised leg		•	•	udhitta padasana / raised leg			•	udhitta padasana / raised leg	•	•	•	udhitta padasana / raised leg		•	•
pavanmuktasana / wind-relieving posture		•	•	anantasana / side-lying leg stretch	•	•	•	tittirasana / partridge		•	•	setu bandhasana / bridge posture	•	•	•
tittirasana / partridge			•	pavanmuktasana / wind-relieving posture	•	•	•	pavanmuktasana / wind-relieving posture	•	•	•	matsyasana / fish posture			•
pavanmuktasana / wind-relieving posture			•	makrasana / crocodile	•	•	•	sasamgasana / hare posture			•	pavanmuktasana / wind-relieving posture	•	•	•
makrasana / crocodile			•	bhujangasana / cobra		•	•	balasana / child's posture			•	adho mukha svanasana / downward-facing dog posture	•	•	•
bilikasana / cat posture	•	•	•	balasana / child's posture		•	•	adho mukha svanasana / downward-facing dog posture		•	•	balasana / child's posture	•	•	•
balasana / child's posture	•	•	•	dandasana / staff posture	•	•	•	balasana / child's posture		•	•	bhujangasana / cobra		•	•
vajrasana / thunderbolt posture	•	•	•	paripurna navasana / complete boat posture			•	dandasana / staff posture			•	balasana / child's posture		•	•
parivrtta vajrasana / thunderbolt twist		•	•	janu sirasana / head-to-knee forward bend		•	•	paschimottanasana / forward bend in sitting	•	•	•	gomukhasana / cow-face posture		•	
vajrasana / thunderbolt posture	•	•	•	baddha konasana / cobbler posture	•	•	•	sukhasana / easy posture	•	•	•	siddhasana / perfect posture	•	•	•
savasana / corpse posture	•	•	•	savasana / corpse posture	•	•	•	savasana / corpse posture	•	•	•	savasana / corpse posture	•	•	•

beginner-level program

The postures selected here are beginner-level. Refer to Part 2 of the book for details on positioning of each posture. With routine practice, the session should be carried out with fluidity and agility of movement. Rest after every posture and steady the breath.

session 1

start

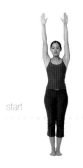

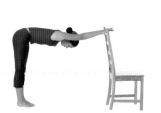

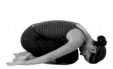

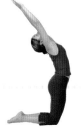

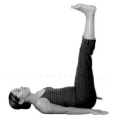

urdhva hastottasana	ardha uttanasana	nagasana	balasana	udhitta padasana
upstretched arms posture	**half standing forward bend**	**raised serpent posture**	**child's posture**	**raised leg posture**
page 40	page 77	page 83	page 56	page 93

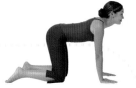

pavanmuktasana	tittirasana	pavanmuktasana	makrasana	bilikasana
wind-relieving posture	**partridge posture**	**wind-relieving posture**	**crocodile posture**	**cat posture**
page 92	page 95	page 92	page 65	pages 52–53

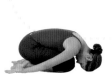

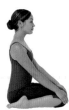

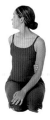

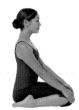

finish

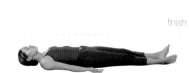

balasana	vajrasana	parivrtta vajrasana	vajrasana	savasana
child's posture	**thunderbolt posture**	**thunderbolt twist**	**thunderbolt posture**	**corpse posture**
page 56	page 51	page 112	page 51	page 91

session 2

start

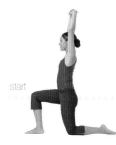

hanumanasana
hanuman posture
page 42

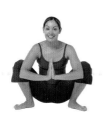

utkatasana
squatting posture
page 41

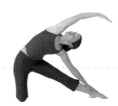

parighasana
cross-bar posture
page 54-55

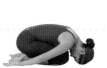

balasana
child's posture
page 56

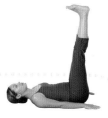

udhitta padasana
raised leg posture
page 93

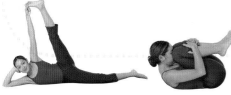

anantasana
side-lying leg raise
page 94

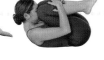

pavanmuktasana
wind-relieving posture
page 92

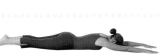

makrasana
crocodile posture
page 65

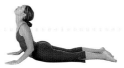

bhujangasana
cobra posture
page 73

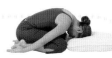

balasana
child's posture
page 56

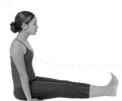

dandasana
staff posture
page 58

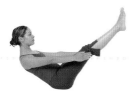

paripurna navasana
complete boat posture
page 61

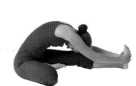

janu sirasana
head-to-knee posture
page 88

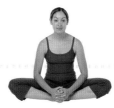

baddha konasana
cobbler posture
page 60

finish

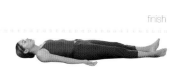

savasana
corpse posture
page 91

session 3

start

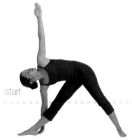

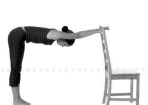

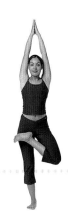

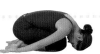

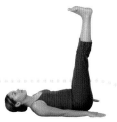

uttihita trikonasana
extended triangle posture
page 43

ardha uttanasana
half standing forward bend
page 77

vrksasana
tree posture
page 102

balasana
child's posture
page 56

udhitta padasana
raised leg posture
page 93

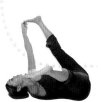

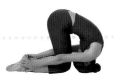

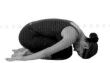

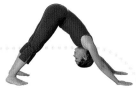

tittirasana
partridge posture
page 95

pavanmuktasana
wind-relieving posture
page 92

sasamgasana
hare posture
page 57

balasana
child's posture
page 56

adho mukha svanasana
downward-facing dog posture
page 66

finish

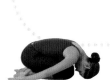

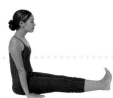

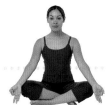

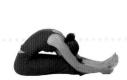

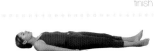

balasana
child's posture
page 56

dandasana
staff posture
page 58

paschimottanasana
forward bend in sitting
page 87

sukhasana
easy posture
page 27

savasana
corpse posture
page 91

session 4

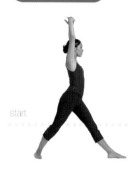

start

virabhadrasana
warrior posture
page 47

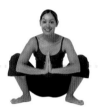

uttanasana
standing forward bend
page 78

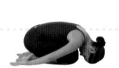

utkatasana
squatting posture
page 41

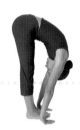

balasana
child's posture
page 56

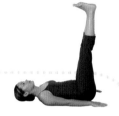

udhitta padasana
raised leg posture
page 93

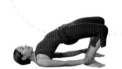

setu bandhasana
bridge posture
page 96

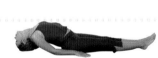

matsyasana
fish posture
page 97

pavanmuktasana
wind-relieving posture
page 92

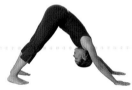

adho mukha svanasana
downward-facing dog posture
page 66

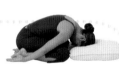

balasana
child's posture
page 56

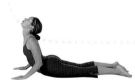

bhujangasana
cobra posture
page 73

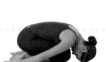

balasana
child's posture
page 56

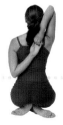

gomukhasana
cow-face posture
page 59

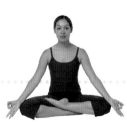

siddhasana
perfect posture
page 62

finish

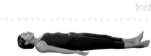

savasana
corpse posture
page 91

for home practice

This is a progressive program of four sessions graded at the intermediate level. When all the postures in the beginner's program can be held with ease, then the intermediate program can be followed. As in the beginner's program, each intermediate-level session can last twenty, thirty, or forty minutes. The postures to be included in each time frame are marked out in Table 2. To progress through the sessions, practice holding the postures for longer. In time, the number of postures carried out in a session can be reduced. As familiarity with the intermediate-level postures increases, the sessions can be adapted to suit your individual needs. The selection of postures for a session should ideally include a spinal twist, a forward bend, an inversion, and a relaxation posture. The Sun salutation is an excellent cycle to begin with, particularly if the session is carried out in the morning.

advisory notes

- Practice in a quiet and well-ventilated room.

- Always spend a few minutes carrying out warm-up exercises (pages 34–37) to prepare all the muscles.

- Be attentive to the exact position of limbs, head, trunk, etc., to attain the correct posture.

- Unless stipulated, breathing should be carried out through the nostrils.

- When a posture is difficult, try the beginner's variation or another similar posture.

- The programs can be adapted to suit individual needs.

- Focus inwardly and work with the breath; allow the body to be stretched to its full potential.

- Wherever possible, carry out the counterpose to each posture.

- Seek medical advice if pain or discomfort is experienced when practicing yoga.

table 2 intermediate-level program

session 1	duration (min) 20	30	40	session 2	duration (min) 20	30	40	session 3	duration (min) 20	30	40	session 4	duration (min) 20	30	40
warm-up exercises	●	●	●	warm-up exercises	●	●	●	warm-up exercises	●	●	●	warm-up exercises	●	●	●
surya namaskar sun salutation (1 cycle)	●	●	●	surya namaskar sun salutation (2 cycles)	●	●	●	surya namaskar sun salutation (4 cycles)	●	●	●	surya namaskar sun salutation (2 cycles)	●	●	●
uttihita trikoasana extended triangle posture	●	●	●	virabhadrasana warrior posture	●	●	●	utthita parsvakonasana extended lateral angle stretch	●	●	●	virabhadrasana cycle	●	●	●
parivrtta trikoasana reverse triangle posture		●	●	ardha chandrasana half moon posture		●	●	uttha chakrasana standing wheel posture		●	●	utthita hasta padangusthasana extended hand-to-big-toe posture			●
uttanasana standing forward bend	●	●	●	uttanasana standing forward bend	●	●	●	uttanasana standing forward bend	●	●	●	parsvottanasana sideways forward stretch	●	●	●
utkatasana chair posture	●	●	●	balasana child's posture	●	●	●	utkatasana chair posture	●	●	●	balasana child's posture	●	●	●
vrksasana tree posture			●	ustrasana camel posture			●	natrajasana dancer posture			●	anjaneyasana crescent moon posture			●
pavanmuktasana wind-relieving posture			●	balasana child's posture			●	pavanmuktasana wind-relieving posture			●	balasana child's posture			●
setu bandhasana bridge posture	●	●	●	sarvangasana shoulder stand			●	sarvangasana shoulder stand		●	●	chakrasana wheel posture		●	●
pavanmuktasana wind-relieving posture	●	●	●	halasana plow posture	●	●	●	karnapidasana ear-closing posture	●	●	●	pavanmuktasana wind-relieving posture		●	●
paripurna navasana complete boat posture	●	●	●	matsyasana fish posture	●	●	●	matsyasana fish posture	●	●	●	ardha sirshasana half headstand	●	●	●
udhitta padasana raised leg posture			●	pavanmuktasana wind-relieving posture	●	●	●	pavanmuktasana wind-relieving posture	●	●	●	balasana child's posture	●	●	●
supta vajrasana supine thunderbolt posture		●	●	bhujangasana cobra posture	●	●	●	salabhasana locust posture		●	●	dhanurasana bow posture		●	●
balasana child's posture		●	●	balasana child's posture		●	●	balasana child's posture	●	●	●	balasana child's posture	●	●	●
vajrasana thunderbolt posture	●	●	●	siddhasana perfect posture	●	●	●	padmasana lotus posture	●	●	●	padmasana lotus posture	●	●	●
savasana corpse posture	●	●	●	savasana corpse posture	●	●	●	savasana corpse posture	●	●	●	savasana corpse posture	●	●	●

intermediate-level program

The postures selected are at the intermediate/advanced level. Particular attention needs to be paid to precise positioning of the body. Take a rest or pause between each posture to harmonize the breath and note the effects on the body.

session 1

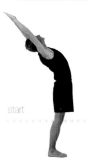

start

surya namaskar
sun salutation (one cycle)

pages 140–141

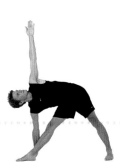

uttihita trikokonasana
extended triangle posture

page 43

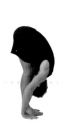

parivrtta trikonasana
reverse triangle posture

page 44

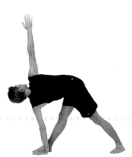

uttanasana
standing forward bend

page 78

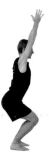

utktatasana
chair posture

page 41

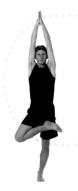

vrksasana
tree posture

page 102

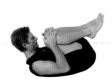

pavanmuktasana
wind-relieving posture

page 92

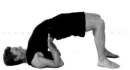

setu bandhasana
bridge posture

page 96

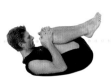

pavanmuktasana
wind-relieving posture

page 92

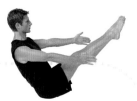

paripurna navasana
complete boat posture

page 61

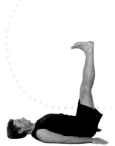

udhitta padasana
raised leg posture

page 93

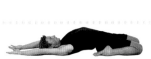

supta vajrasana
supine thunderbolt posture

page 84

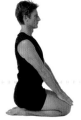

balasana
child's posture

page 56

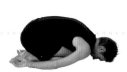

vajrasana
thunderbolt posture

page 51

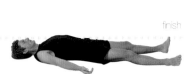

finish

savasana
corpse posture

page 91

session 2

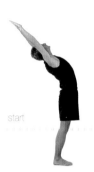
start

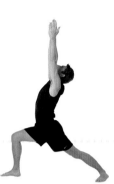

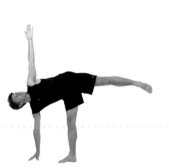

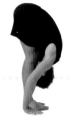

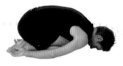

surya namaskar
sun salutation (two cycles)
pages 140–141

virabhadrasana
warrior posture
page 47

ardha chandrasana
half moon posture
page 106

uttanasana
standing forward bend
page 78

balasana
child's posture
page 56

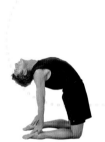

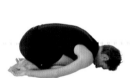

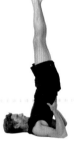

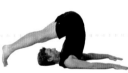

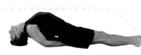

ustrasana
camel posture
page 85

balasana
child's posture
page 56

sarvangasana
shoulder stand
page 117

halasana
plow posture
pages 118–119

matsyasana
fish posture
page 97

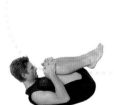

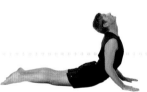

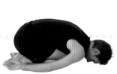

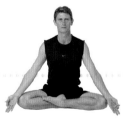

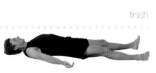
finish

pavanmuktasana
wind-relieving posture
page 92

bhujangasana
cobra posture
page 73

balasana
child's posture
page 56

siddhasana
perfect posture
page 62

savasana
corpse posture
page 91

session 3

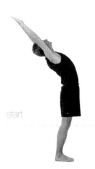

start

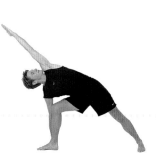

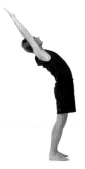

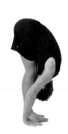

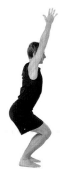

surya namaskar
sun salutation (four cycles)

pages 140–141

utthita parsvakonasana
extended lateral angle stretch

page 45

uttha chakrasana
standing wheel posture

page 81

uttanasana
standing forward bend

page 78

sahaj utkatasana
chair pose

page 41

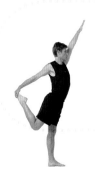

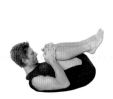

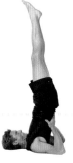

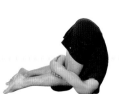

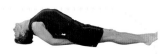

natrajasana
dancer posture

page 103

pavanmuktasana
wind-relieving posture

page 92

sarvangasana
shoulder stand

page 117

karnapidasana
ear-closing posture

page 120

matsyasana
fish posture

page 97

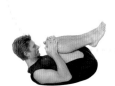

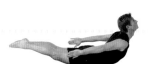

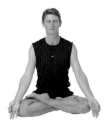

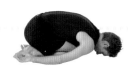

finish

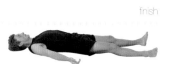

pavanmuktasana
wind-relieving posture

page 92

salabhasana
locust posture

pages 70–71

balasana
child's posture

page 56

padmasana
lotus posture

page 63

savasana
corpse posture

page 91

session 4

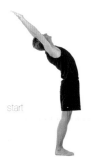

start

surya namaskar
sun salutation (two cycles)

pages 140–141

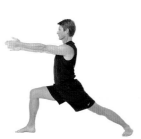

virabhadrasana cycle

pages 48–49

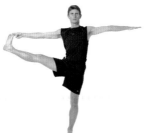

utthita hasta padangusthasana
extended hand-to-big-toe posture

page 105

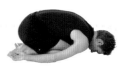

parsvottanasana
sideways forward stretch

page 80

balasana
child's posture

page 56

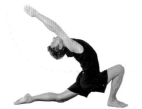

anjaneyasana
crescent moon posture

page 86

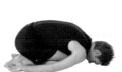

balasana
child's posture

page 56

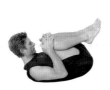

chakrasana
wheel posture

page 98

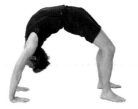

pavanmuktasana
wind-relieving posture

page 92

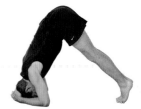

ardha sirshasana
half headstand

page 121

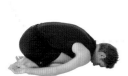

balasana
child's posture

page 56

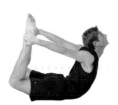

dhanurasana
bow posture

pages 74–75

balasana
child's posture

page 56

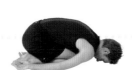

padmasana
lotus posture

page 63

finish

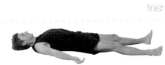

savasana
corpse posture

page 91

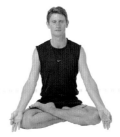

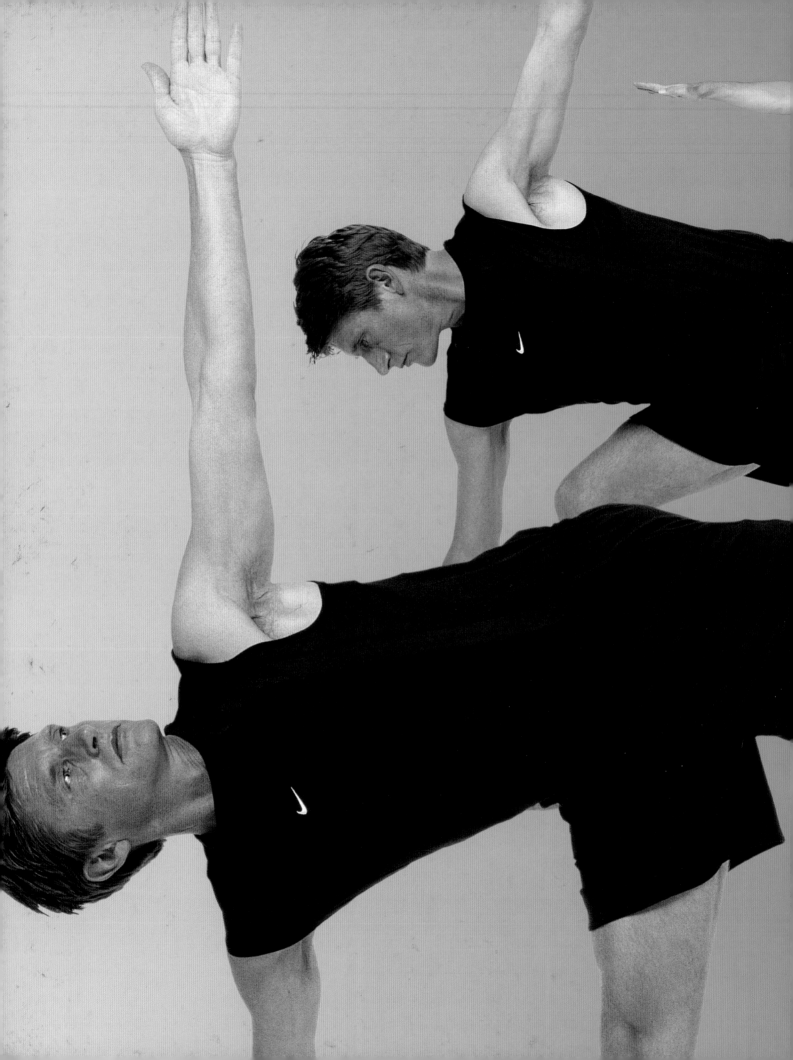

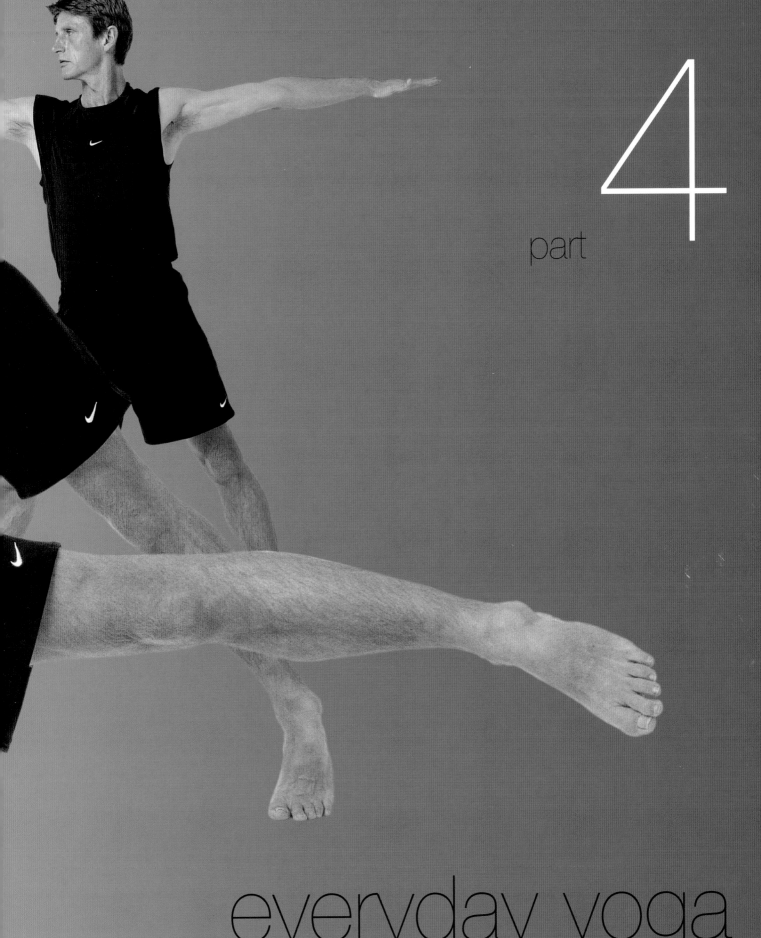

part 4

everyday yoga

surya namaskar **sun salutation**

Surya namaskar, or the Sun salutation, is a beautiful greeting to our glorious sun, the source of all life on earth. It is traditionally performed at dawn, facing east, when the cosmic energy, or *prana,* is considered to be high.

Surya namaskar is a sequence of twelve positions performed gracefully one after the other in a flowing cycle. Each position counteracts the one before and is synchronized with inhalations and exhalations. For beginners, it will be some time before the cycle flows smoothly. At whatever level, the practice of Surya namaskar brings enormous benefits. It increases spinal flexibility, limbers up the joints, regulates the breath, and focuses the mind in preparation for asanas.

benefits • Improves circulation • Improves general muscle tone • Stimulates the nervous system • Reduces psychosomatic tension

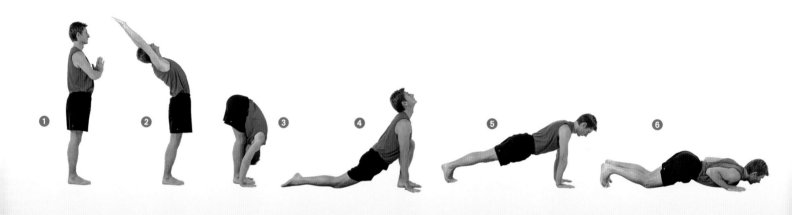

❶ Stand in Tadasana (page 39). Bring the palms together in prayer position in front of the chest with the fingers pointing upward. Look straight ahead. Hold for two to three breathing cycles and visualize the image of the sun rising above the horizon and revitalizing every cell of the body. Exhale.

❷ Inhaling deeply, draw the arms up, bending backward from the waist, pushing the hips out, and keeping the legs straight. The head should be between the arms and the span of the hands widens as the arms are raised.

❸ Exhaling, bend forward from the hips. Relax at the neck. Keep the legs straight and either place the palms flat or rest the fingertips on the floor, beside the feet. If the hands cannot reach the floor, then bend the knees. The hands stay in this position for the next several moves.

❹ Inhaling, stretch the right leg back. Rest the knee on the floor, arch the back, and turn the face upward.

❺ Retain the breath as both feet are brought together so that the legs, back, and head are in an inclined plane. Look at the floor.

❻ Exhaling, lower the knees onto the floor. Then lower the chest and forehead to rest on the floor. Keep the toes turned in, the hips off the floor, and the elbows close to the body. (This is the position known as *Ashtanga namaskar,* or "Eightfold salutation," as eight parts of the body are touching the floor.)

O life giving Sun, offspring of the Lord of Creation, solitary seer of heaven! Spread thy light and withdraw thy blinding splendor that I may behold thy radiant form: That Spirit far away within thee is my own inmost Spirit.

Isopanishad

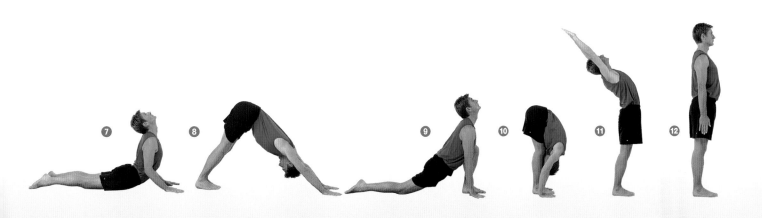

❼ Inhaling, lower the hips, turn the toes away, and raise the chest and head. Turn to look up. Relax the abdomen and legs. (This is *Bhujangasana,* or the Cobra posture.)

❽ Exhaling, turn the toes in and raise the hips high so that the body assumes an inverted *V* shape. The back should be as straight as possible and the heels pressed downward. Relax the neck and look at the toes. (This is *Adho mukha svanasana,* or the Downward-facing dog posture.)

❾ Inhaling deeply, bring the right leg forward, lining up the toes with the fingers. Rest the knee on the floor, arch the back, and turn the face upward. Press the palms and right foot down to fix in place. (This position is the same as position 4, but with the opposite leg forward.)

❿ Exhaling, bring the left leg forward and align with the right foot and fingers. (This is the same as position 3.)

⓫ Inhaling deeply, straighten to a standing position. Draw the arms up, bending backward from the waist, pushing the hips out and keeping legs straight. (This is the same as position 2.)

⓬ Exhaling, lower the arms with the palms pressed together. Return the hands to the side of the body to return to Tadasana, poised to begin another cycle. To balance the body, lead with the left leg, this time from position 4.

In the beginning, two to three cycles of Surya namaskar are ample. With practice, build up to six to twelve cycles.

morning wake-up routine (30 minutes)

On awakening and rising from bed, many of us naturally stretch by extending the arms and hands, legs and feet, and arching the spine. This fulfills the body's natural yearning to be stretched out after several hours of inactivity. Yoga asanas performed early in the morning are simply an extension of the body's need to be stretched, but in a more disciplined and effective manner.

The early morning period, shortly after awakening, is an ideal time to practice yoga. The cosmic energy is said to be high, and the body, having rested through the night, is able to sustain the postures for longer periods. However, the body is generally stiffer in the morning than in the evening, so warm-up exercises must be used to prepare the muscles for asanas. In towns and cities, the pollution level has dropped, making the morning an optimal time to practice deeper breathing. The asanas should ideally be performed after emptying the bladder and bowels and having a bath or shower. This morning practice will have a very beneficial effect on the body's energy levels throughout the day.

Begin by lying in Savasana for one minute.

warm-ups: Neck stretch, Upper arm stretch, Hip rotation, Thigh stretch, Knee-to-head in supine position, Surya namaskar, Sun salutation (one cycle), Warrior cycle (one cycle)

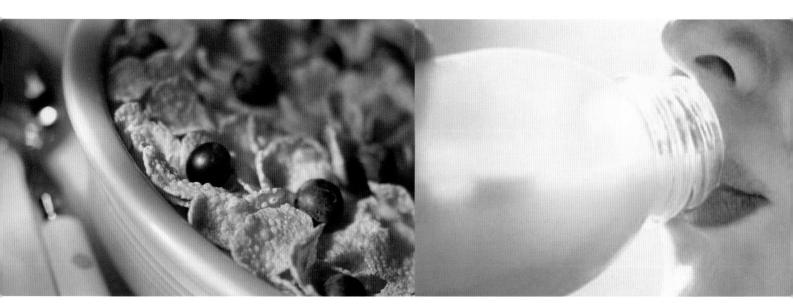

energize yourself

Breakfast is the most important meal of the day, and it's crucial that you don't skip it. Remember, it's been at least eight hours since you last ate. So once you've completed your morning yoga routine, make sure you sit down and take the time to fuel your body ready for the day ahead. Here are a couple of healthy breakfast suggestions:

summer

Fresh fruit juice or lemon, honey, and water drink
Yogurt, fresh fruit, dates, and honey

winter

Green tea
Cereal or oatmeal
Toasted whole-grain bread
Fruit

making time for yoga

Planning your routine more effectively would enable time for yoga practice. Organize yourself going to bed, preparing the contents of the workbag or briefcase, selecting an outfit, making sandwiches. Most people need eight hours of uninterrupted sleep. This does reduce for some people with age. Make sure that you do get your needed sleep quota. Rushing around in the morning simply sets the pattern of feeling stressed throughout the day.

above left: Cereal is a quick, healthy option for the day's most important meal, breakfast.
above right: The vitamin C in orange juice starts the day off well.

breathing exercises

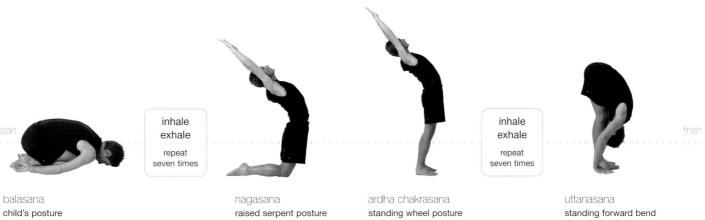

start

balasana
child's posture

page 56

inhale
exhale

repeat
seven times

nagasana
raised serpent posture

page 83

ardha chakrasana
standing wheel posture

page 81

inhale
exhale

repeat
seven times

uttanasana
standing forward bend

page 78

finish

postures

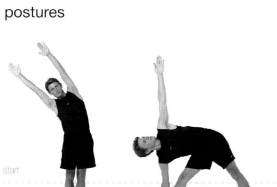 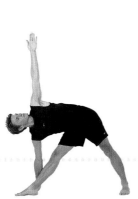 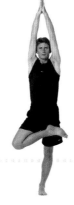 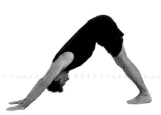 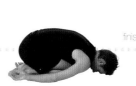

start

urdhva hastottasana
upstretched arms posture

page 40

uttihita trikonasana
extended triangle posture

page 43

vrkasana
tree posture

page 102

mukha svanasana
downward-facing dog posture

page 66

balasana
child's posture

page 56

finish

intermediate level can replace or follow with:

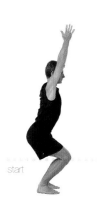 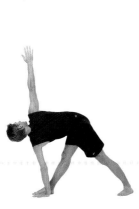 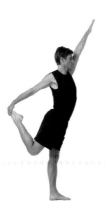 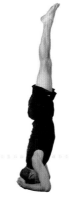 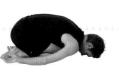

start

sahaj utkatasana
chair posture

page 41

parivrtta trikonsana
reverse triangle posture

page 44

natarajasana
dancer posture

page 103

ardha sirshasana or sirshasana
half headstand or headstand

pages 121–122

balasana
child's posture

page 56

finish

dynamic energizing routine (20 minutes)

Asanas can be performed in two ways. Static practice is when the asanas are held for a certain period. The focus is on the breath and extending the area of the body that the asana focuses on. Dynamic practice is when the body moves in and out of the asana with the rhythmic inhalation and exhalation of the breath. Dynamic practice often involves moving in and out of an asana and its counterasana. For individuals who are used to undertaking aerobic exercises, this is a good way of learning the yoga asanas and preparing for static practice, which is considered to be more difficult to achieve. The rhythmic movements of tensing and relaxing different muscle groups generates heat and prepares the muscles for static practice. The dynamic practice of a yoga asana brings new insight into the possibilities of the asana. It increases awareness of the muscles being used and how the breath can be used to explore the posture. It is a valuable way for both beginners and experienced students to practice.

warm-ups: Woodcutter, Sun salutation (2 cycles)

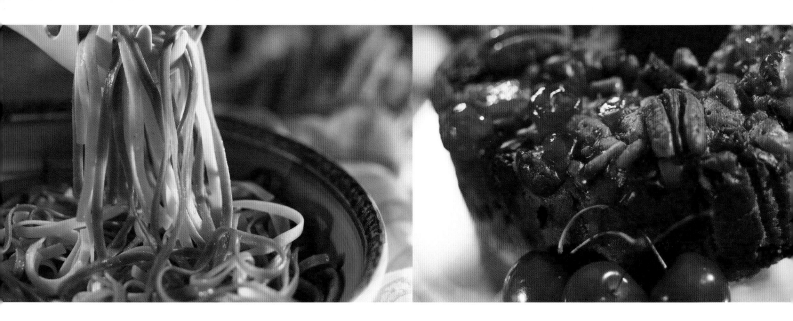

Follow this exercise routine with one of these wholesome snacks:

summer
Fresh fruit juice with sliced strawberries
Hummus and pita bread with bean-sprout salad

winter
Lemon tea with a slice of fresh lime
Vegetable soup with whole-grain bread
Banana, yogurt, and honey

Other ways to increase your energy levels are:
• Ginseng is considered a great natural energy booster, so try ginseng tea as an alternative to caffeinated tea or coffee.
• Have a regular bedtime routine. The biggest cause of lack of energy is disturbed sleep. Even if you can't get a good eight hours' sleep each night, at least try to make sure you're going to bed at the same time each evening.
• Watch out for refined sugar. It can give you a quick "high" of energy, but will later make you feel sluggish.
• Avoid heavy meals that include a lot of bread, pasta, or dairy products. If you want to be alert, you don't want to eat too much of these foods—they'll send you to sleep!
• Enjoy what you're doing! Try to include an activity that you like among your duties. Your natural interest will spark your energy levels.

above left: Eat too much bulky food, such as pasta, and your energy levels will suffer.
above right: The refined sugar in cakes and sweets will only give you a temporary rush of energy.

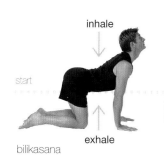

start

inhale

exhale

bilikasana
cat posture

pages 52–53

inhale
exhale

repeat
seven times

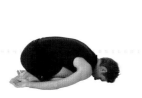

balasana
child's posture

page 56

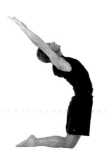

nagasana
raised serpent posture

page 83

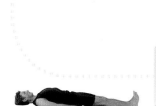

savasana
corpse posture

page 91

inhale
exhale

repeat
seven times

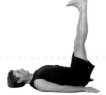

udhitta padasana
raised leg posture

page 93

inhale
exhale

repeat
seven times

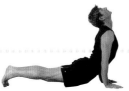

urdhva mukha svanasana
upward-facing dog posture

page 67

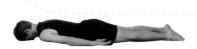

lying in prone position

page 65

inhale
exhale

repeat
seven times

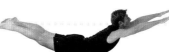

dolasana
swing posture

page 72

finish

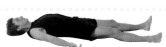

savasana
corpse posture

page 91

lunchtime refocusing routine **(15 minutes)**

When the mind is engaged on a task, it can be difficult to disengage. People in the office can spend long hours in front of the computer, on the telephone, or writing at the desk. When deadlines need to be achieved and the pace of work is fast, mental weariness can rapidly set in. Sitting at a desk for long periods can cause stiffness in the joints, rounded shoulders, poor posture, tired eyes, and shallow breathing. All these things can have a detrimental effect on concentration and performance. Making good use of the lunch break by spending a few minutes stretching the muscles with yoga asanas can have an immensely beneficial effect on concentration and focus. Recharge, refocus, and reflect with yoga asanas to enhance performance and reinvigorate your approach to a work task or problem.

This program comprises warm-up exercises that can be carried out from standing or sitting on a chair. Find a secluded corner in the workplace to carry out the asanas. The program contains standing or kneeling asanas, which require very little floor space.

warm-ups: Neck stretch, Shoulder rolls, Upper arm stretch, Sitting arm and neck stretch, Front-to-side leg raise, and Thigh stretch

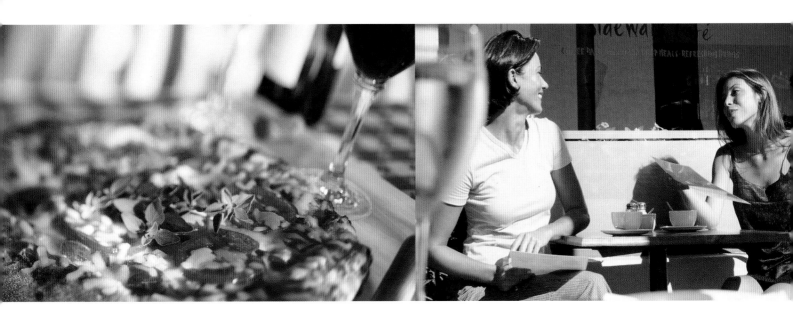

Lunchtime is your opportunity to replenish your body and get ready for the rest of the day, so take advantage of it.

healthy eating

Try to avoid eating a heavy lunch. It's much better to have small snacks during the course of the day than to starve yourself and then overcompensate with a huge sandwich. Overeating will make you very drowsy in the afternoon. Try to stick to healthier alternatives. Cut down on the coffee and drink green tea instead (it has several beneficial properties), make sure you eat some fresh vegetables or fruit, and choose whole-grain bread. You'll feel much better for it!

take a hike

Don't waste your lunch hour sitting at your desk. Even if it's only for ten minutes, try to get out of the office for a short walk. It's important to get out, get some fresh air, and mentally walk away from your work for a short while at least.

above left: Heavy eating at lunchtime will kill your afternoon energy levels.
above right: It's important to get out of your working environment at lunchtime.

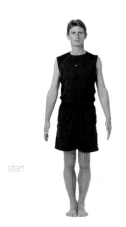

tadasana
mountain posture
page 39

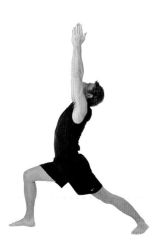

virabhadrasana
warrior posture
page 47

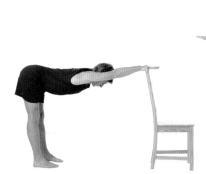

ardha uttanasana
standing half forward bend
page 77

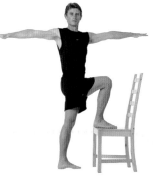

maricyasana
standing spinal twist
page 109

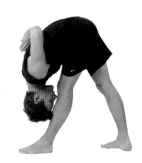

parsvottanasana
sideways forward stretch
page 80

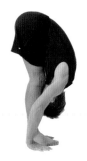

uttanasana
standing forward bend
page 78

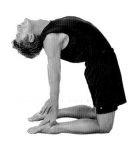

ustrasana
camel posture
page 85

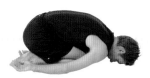

balasana
child's posture
page 56

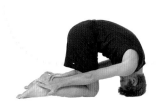

sasamgasana
hare posture
page 57

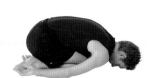

balasana
child's posture
page 56

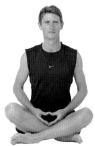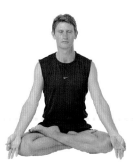

Complete the session with sitting in Sukhasana (page 27) or Padmasana (page 63) for two to three minutes with eyes closed. Focus on deepening and lengthening the breath.

relaxing bedtime routine (20 minutes)

After an active day, where many different events have occurred, the mind may be in a whirl of thoughts. The muscles can hold on to tension and the joints may feel stiff. Yoga performed before the night's sleep is a great way to unwind, release tension, and relax the body. This relaxing bedtime routine will promote a peaceful and restive sleep.

warm-ups: Neck stretch, Shoulder rolls, Rocking the body

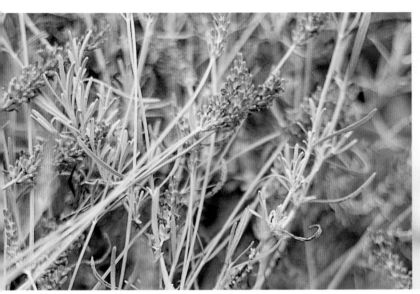 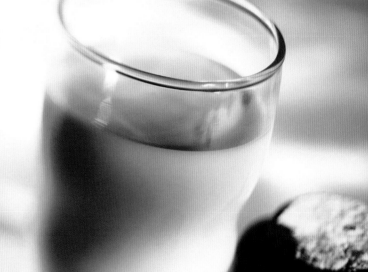

As well as yoga exercises, there are a number of other ways you can make sure you get a good night's sleep:

hot bath

Taking a hot bath as soon as you get in from work is a wonderful way of winding down at the end of the day. Not only does the warm water help your muscles relax, your mind is allowed to slowly unwind as well. Up to six drops of lavender oil added to the bathwater will help you relax further.

comfortable clothes

Once out of the bath, climb into comfortable clothes—preferably cotton—to help yourself feel as relaxed as possible. There's nothing better than slinking around the house in a pair of pajamas!

call it a day

A couple of hours before you intend to go to bed, start to cut out all stimulants. Try switching the television off in favor of a book, don't eat anything, and avoid alcohol (though a glass of milk is a good idea). Take the phone off the hook and switch off the computer. All of this helps your mind and body get used to the idea that the day is over.

above left: Lavender essential oils aid relaxation.
above right: A glass of milk at the end of the day will help you go to sleep.

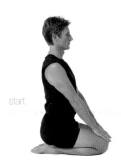

start

vajrasana
thunderbolt posture

page 51

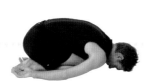

balasana
child's posture

page 56

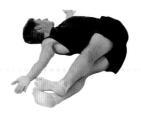

jathara parivartanasana
belly-turning posture

pages 114–115

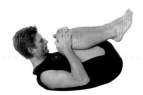

pavanmuktasana
wind-relieving posture

page 92

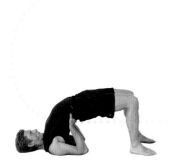

setu bandhasana
bridge posture

page 96

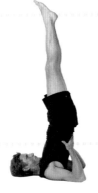

sarvangasana
shoulder stand

page 117

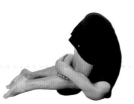

karnapidasana
ear-closing posture

page 120

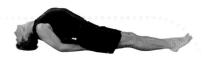

matsyasana
fish posture

page 97

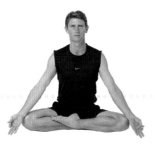

siddhasana
breathing in perfect posture

page 62

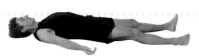

finish

savasana
corpse posture

page 91

routines for women (10 minutes)

Women often find it difficult to take time out to focus on themselves in today's fast-paced and challenging world. The woman who gets fatigued or stressed may find herself unable to carry out the activities that she planned to do in leisure time. Dedicating just ten minutes to practicing yoga will balance the hormones, harmonize the mind and body, and increase energy levels. The programs here are specifically tailored to benefit women at different stages of their lives.

routine for premenstrual syndrome (PMS)

warm-ups: Upper arm stretch, Sitting arm and neck stretch, Front-to-side leg raise and Thigh stretch (pages 34–37)

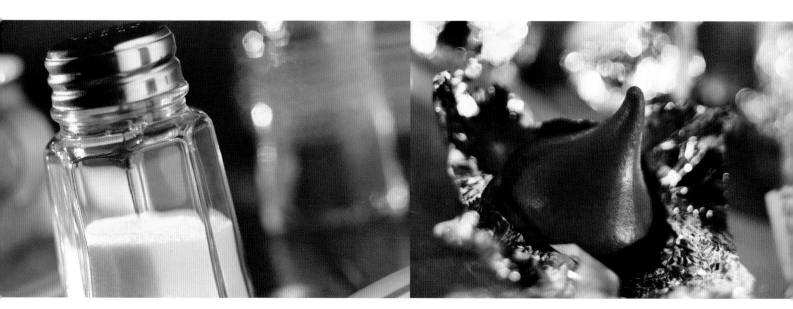

Premenstrual syndrome refers to the collection of physical and emotional symptoms that precede the onset of the period. PMS is experienced to one degree or another by some 70 percent of women. The physical symptoms include tenderness of the breasts, general fluid retention, fatigue, abdominal bloating, and joint pains in the legs. The emotional symptoms include aggressiveness, irritability, and tearfulness. If the symptoms are severe, then consult your medical practitioner. The gentle stretching experienced through yoga helps to massage the internal organs and improve blood circulation. This assists in improving the function of hormone-producing glands and hormonal imbalances are harmonized. The calming and relaxing effects of yoga will help to stabilize the emotions.

above left: It's best to keep away from salt during PMS.
above right: The body often craves chocolate before menstruation.

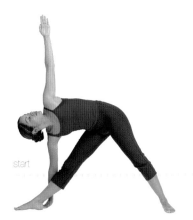

start

uttihita trikoasana
extended triangle posture

page 43

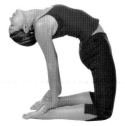

uttanasana
standing forward bend

page 78

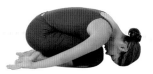

ustrasana
camel posture

page 85

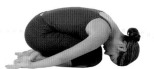

balasana
child's posture

page 56

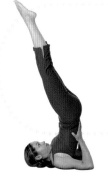

sarvangasana
shoulder stand

page 117

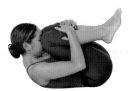

pavanmuktasana
wind-relieving posture

page 92

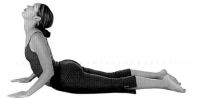

bhujangasana
cobra posture

page 73

balasana
child's posture

page 56

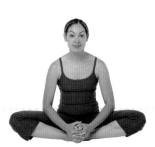

baddha konasana
cobbler posture

(follow with the butterfly posture)

page 60

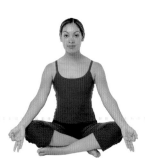

pranayama in sukhasana
breathing in easy posture

page 27

finish

routine after menstruation (to be practiced from day three of the cycle)

warm-ups: Rocking the body (page 37)

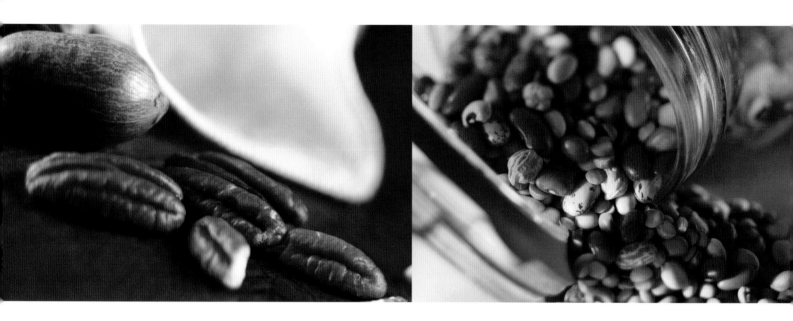

From the onset of puberty to menopause, women experience the cycle of fertility lasting on average twenty-eight days. During the cycle, the ovaries produce an egg, which is deposited at the entrance of the fallopian tube leading into the uterus. If the egg remains unfertilized, estrogen levels drop and trigger the shedding of the blood-rich vascular lining of the womb, beginning the menstrual blood flow. The episode usually lasts between three to five days and involves the loss of about an ounce of blood. During menstruation, women should decrease their physical activity. Relaxation postures are the most suitable yoga positions, though generally all postures should be avoided during the first part of the cycle. When the flow has diminished considerably, usually after the third day of menstruation, then selective yoga postures can be practiced. If the menstrual flow is heavy and lasts for longer then three days, then practice only after the flow has diminished. The gentle stretches, which limber up the pelvis and stretch the lower back and legs, are particularly beneficial at this time.

above left: Nuts are a good source of magnesium, which can help with muscle cramps.
above right: Seeds are rich in vitamin B6, which can help with the symptoms of PMS.

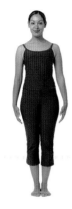

start

tadasana
mountain posture
page 39

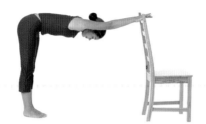
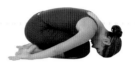

ardha uttansana
half-standing forward bend
page 77

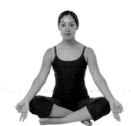

balasana
child's posture
page 56

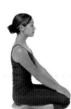

vajrasana
thunderbolt posture
page 51

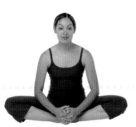

baddha konasana
cobbler posture
(follow with the butterfly posture)
page 60

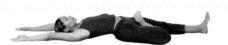

supta vrksasana
supine tree posture
page 99

pranayama in sukhasana
breathing in easy posture
page 27

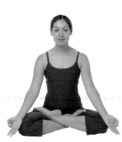

meditation in siddhasana
perfect posture
page 62

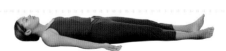

finish

savasana
corpse posture
page 91

routine for menopause

warm-ups: Sitting arm and neck stretch, Head-to-knee in supine, Rocking the body (pages 36–37)

Menopause is a period of emotional and physical change that women undergo when their periods cease. It is a natural process that women experience in their life cycle. Many women readily embrace the postmenopausal stage and welcome the changes. There is no longer concern over pregnancy and PMS. For other women, it can be a distressing period as the changes are seen as a loss of fertility and youth. In some ancient cultures the postmenopausal woman was attributed with wisdom and a spiritual wakening. Postmenopausal women often governed the ancient rites of pagan Ireland, as they were considered to be the wisest of mortals because they permanently retained their wise blood.

Menopause usually occurs around the age of fifty, but for some women periods can cease at forty or as late as sixty. During menopause, the delicate balance of hormonal production of the ovaries, pituitary gland, and hypothalamus is altered. As the body adjusts to diminishing estrogen production, women commonly experience symptoms such as hot flashes and sweating. Women may also experience sleep disturbances, poor concentration, joint pains, frequent urination, vaginal dryness, irritability, and headaches. Only a small proportion of women experience these symptoms to a distressing level.

The gentle stretching of yoga postures massages the internal organs and regulates their function, helping the body to adjust to the physical changes. The breathing exercises and relaxation poses help to calm the mind and mentally prepare for the changes to the body.

self-help

To control the body's temperature, wear several layers of light clothing, preferably high in cotton content, so that they can be easily removed. Sleep in a cool room. Avoid hot baths and take frequent lukewarm showers. Keep a diary of episodes of hot flashes and use this to identify possible triggers and times.

treatment

Some medical practitioners recommend a form of treatment called Hormone Replacement Therapy (HRT). HRT artificially restores hormone levels and reduces the physical symptoms. HRT is also believed to reduce the risk of osteoporosis. However, many gynecologists are concerned about the long-term effects of HRT and recommend that it be discontinued after the age of fifty-five. Evening primrose is thought to be beneficial in regulating the hormones. Vaginal dryness can be soothed by the application of calendula ointment or douching the vagina with yogurt solution. Alternative treatments such as homeopathy are thought to be an effective way of relieving the symptoms of menopause.

dietary considerations

During the onset of menopause, eat food high in calcium, zinc, vitamin E, and vitamin B complex. Eat a high-fiber diet to ensure the digestive system is working efficiently. Avoid tea, coffee, alcohol, and rich, fatty foods, and drink plenty of water and fresh fruit juices.

suggestions for meals

breakfast
- Whole-grain cereal, with fresh strawberries and milk or plain yogurt
- Whole-grain toast with honey
- Oatmeal and raisins, green tea

main meals
- Grilled white fish, green salad
- Mushroom crêpe, couscous salad
- Brown pasta, marinated olives, and arugula salad
- Seed bake, steamed vegetables

desserts
- Whole-grain apple crumble
- Fruit and yogurt
- Brown-rice pudding with raisins
- Baked banana with orange juice

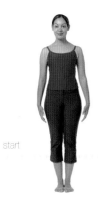

start

tadasana
mountain posture

page 39

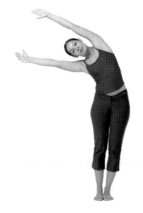

urdhva hastottasana
upstretched arms posture

page 40

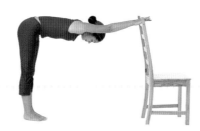

ardha uttanasana
half-standing forward bend

page 77

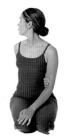

parivrtta vajrasana
thunderbolt twist

page 112

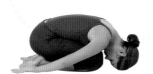

balasana
child's posture

page 56

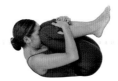

setu bandhasana
bridge posture

page 96

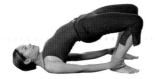

pavanmuktansana
wind-relieving posture

page 92

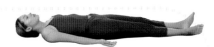

savasana
corpse posture

page 91

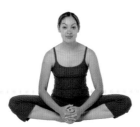

baddha konasana
cobbler posture

(follow with the butterfly posture)

page 60

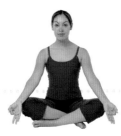

pranayama in sukhasana
breathing in easy posture

page 27

finish

routine for pregnancy (from three to six months)

The postures practiced during pregnancy are dependent on the mother's level of fitness, health, and stage of pregnancy. Because of the very individual needs of the pregnant woman, yoga during pregnancy is best carried out under the guidance of an antenatal yoga teacher. Not all the postures shown here may be suitable for some mothers. The session outline is best used as a guide. If at all unsure of the suitability of a posture, consult a midwife or doctor.

warm-ups: Shoulder rolls, Upper arm stretch, Windmill, Sitting arm and neck stretch (pages 34–36)

Yoga will promote health and improve energy for both mother and child. Yoga postures are an ideal way to prepare the body for the pregnancy and will help build a strong bond between the mother and baby. The postures enable the spine to be strengthened and encourage the lower back to lengthen downward so that the uterus is securely cupped in the pelvis. The baby's weight is borne through the hips and legs rather then the lower back. The postures also allow the baby in the mother's womb to experience different spatial positions. The massaging effect of the stretches on the womb assists the flow of oxygen and nutrients to the baby. The postures selected here will help to alleviate the more common problems of tension and stress.

The sitting postures Baddha konasana and Sukhasana may be suitable for those with no prior experience of yoga. To be comfortable, sit on a folded blanket as this helps to keep the body warm and assists in the leg positions. If maintaining an erect spine is difficult, then sit against a wall. These are also useful positions in which to practice pranayama. Breathing is central to any antenatal yoga program. Pranayama will increase the body's awareness of breathing patterns and help to prepare for the physical changes that pregnancy brings. When carrying out an asana, always move slowly and be guided by the body's needs. After each asana, relax for one to two minutes, either lying on the back or on the side. Make use of blankets and cushions to give support, particularly as the pregnancy advances.

clothing

Through the pregnancy months, a woman's body changes. Wear loose, comfortable clothing made of natural fibers, which do not restrict breathing and allow complete freedom in movements. Ensure that the area around the abdomen is not being compressed.

diet

The pregnancy diet should include a high fiber intake, steamed vegetables, plenty of fresh fruit, dairy products, nuts, dried fruit, and plenty of water. Be intuitive to the body's needs and eat food that the body craves. Have at least three meals a day, chewing the food well. Don't rush the meal.

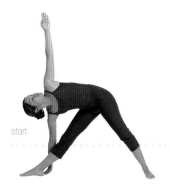

uttihita trikoasana

extended triangle posture

page 43

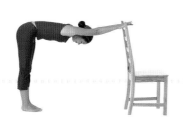

ardha uttanasana

half-standing forward bend

page 77

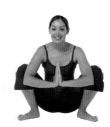

utkatasana

squatting posture

page 41

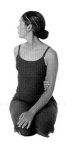

parivrtta vajrasana

thunderbolt twist

page 112

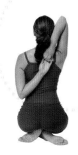

gomukhasana

cow-face posture

page 59

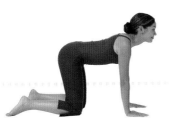

bilikasana

cat posture

pages 52–53

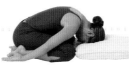

balasana

child's posture

(knees apart and head resting on pillow)

page 56

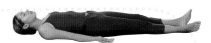

savasana

corpse posture

page 91

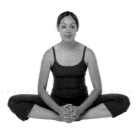

baddha konasana

cobbler posture

(follow with the butterfly posture)

page 60

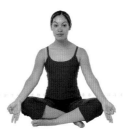

pranayama in sukhasana

breathing in easy posture

page 27

finish

postnatal yoga **(20 minutes)** eight weeks after giving birth

level: Beginner

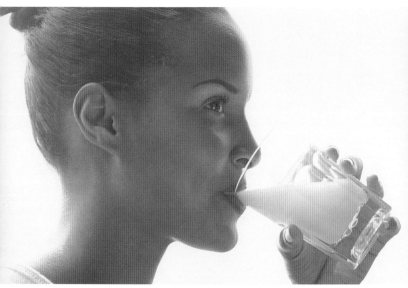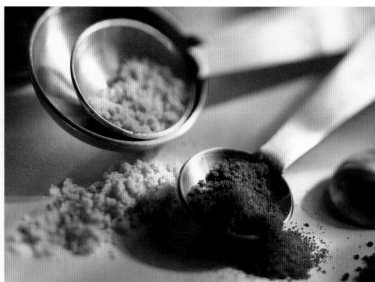

Motherhood is a wonderful experience. Nurturing a newborn baby is very demanding and can be exhausting. After the birth, many women become conscious of excess fat often acquired during pregnancy. Yoga can play an important role in regaining your shape and help you cope with stress and fatigue. Whether the birth was natural or assisted, the focused breathing to promote relaxation can be used from the very first day. Maintaining clarity and calmness will help you contend with the demands of motherhood and establish the unique bond between baby and mother. The cat posture can be performed soon after a natural birth, as it helps the womb return to its normal position. It also helps the muscles of the vagina, if distended during the birth, to regain their original elasticity. Choose a quiet time of the day to practice. Generally, yoga can be practiced eight weeks after an uncomplicated birth and twelve weeks after a complicated birth. Ensure that tears are properly healed before practicing postures and ask your physician about the optimum time for starting yoga.

above left: Try to drink a glass of juice or water each time you breast-feed so that you don't get too deyhdrated.
above right Avoid spicy food if you're breast-feeding, as your new baby may get stomach upset from the strong tastes that are passed on in your milk.

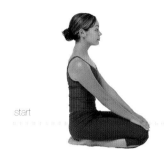

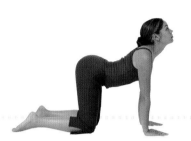

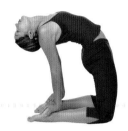

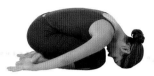

start

vajrasana
thunderbolt posture

page 51

bilikasana
cat posture

pages 52–53

ustrasana
camel posture

page 85

balasana
child's posture

page 56

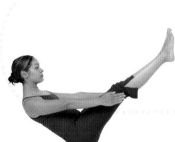

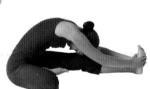

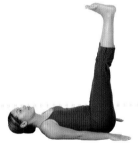

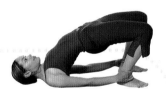

paripurna navasana
complete boat posture

page 61

janu sirsasana
head-to-knee posture

page 88

udhitta padasana
raised leg posture

page 93

setu bandhasana
bridge posture

page 96

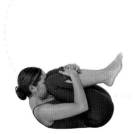

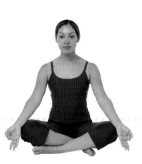

finish

pavanmuktasana
wind-relieving posture

page 92

sukhasana
easy posture

page 27

Complete the session with sitting in Sukhasana (page 27) or
Padmasana (page 63) for 2–3 minutes with eyes closed. Focus
on deepening and lengthening the breath.

toning and slimming yoga for the body

All yoga asanas have a multitude of beneficial effects. Each asana is cleverly designed to address different parts of the body, stretching and toning various muscle groups and nourishing specific internal organs or systems. Many asanas work to regulate the metabolic rate and eliminate toxins from the body. Yoga asanas improve energy levels, calm the mind, tone the muscles, and bring youthfulness and poise to the body. For the body that carries excess fat, many of the yoga asanas may at first be difficult to attain comfortably. However, with diligent practice and perseverance, asanas that balance out the internal systems as well as tone the muscles will also reduce excess fat.

In the figure opposite, asanas listed are linked to the body part that is strongly stretched.

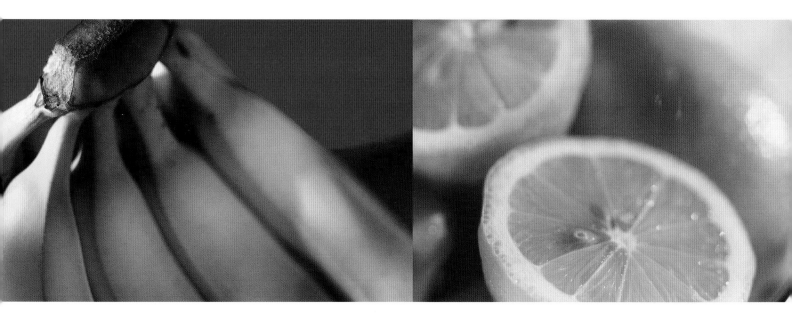

Many asanas work on nourishing specific internal organs or systems and help to regulate the metabolic rate and eliminate toxins from the body. Sarvangasana and sirshasana are two postures that are thought to assist weight reduction. While holding in Sarvangasana, the metabolic rate is believed to double. The regular practice of Sirshasana is thought to reduce the size of the stomach and hence regulate appetite. Yoga asanas improve energy levels, calm the mind, and bring youthfulness and poise to the body. As the practice of yoga brings vitality and serenity into your life, harmful habits such as smoking, alcohol consumption, and overeating will no longer be compatible and will be effortlessly discarded. The overconsumption of food is often linked to an emotional need. Relaxation and breathing exercises, which are so beneficial for calming the mind, will help to break any overattachment to food.

simple guidelines for healthy eating
● Drink lots of water—two-thirds of your body is made up of water. Water is an essential body requirement for maintaining healthy cells and removing toxins from the body. Drink water throughout the day.

Get into the habit of carrying water wherever you go and use this to quench your thirst. Decrease the intake of diuretics such as tea and coffee, which actually decrease the fluid in the cells.
● Eat natural foods—avoid refined foods that are likely to have a high fat, sugar, or salt content. A good way of reducing the intake of toxins is to eat an organic diet. Fresh fruit and raw vegetables in salads provide the minerals and vitamins that our bodies need.
● Try fasting for a day—to cleanse the internal systems, eat only fruits and drink lots of water and fruit juices. Do not fast if pregnant or breast-feeding.
● Eat smaller meals—food should be consumed according to the body's requirements. Practicing yoga postures is a good way of regulating the body's needs.
● Chew your food well—the breakdown of food begins in the mouth. By chewing meals well, the body is able to derive the nutrition from a smaller intake of food. Sit at the table and take your time over a meal. Experience and enjoy the meal.

above left and right: Fresh fruit can be a good source of fiber, vitamins, and potassium.

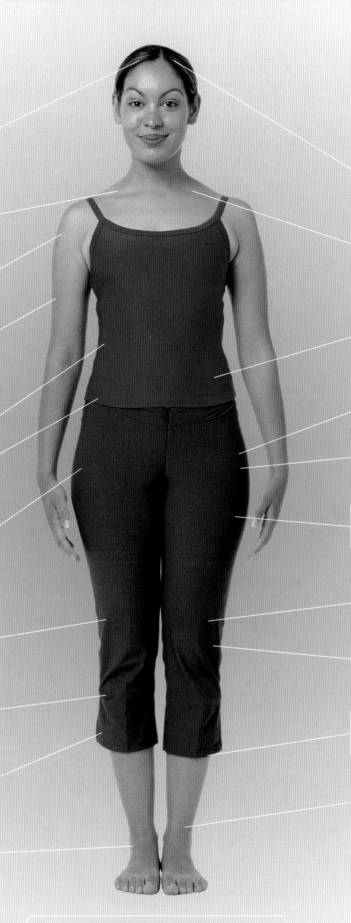

ardha sirshasana
half headstand

sirshasana **headstand**
(reduces the size of the stomach,
hence regulating appetite)

matsyasana
fish posture

anjaneyasana
crescent moon posture

nagasana
raised serpent posture

ustrasana
camel posture

gomukhasana
cow-face posture

chakrasana
wheel posture

urdhva hastottasana
upstretched arms posture

paripurna navasana
complete boat posture

bhujangasana
cobra posture

jathara parivartanasana
belly turning posture

setu bandhasana
bridge posture

dhanurasana
bow posture

tittirasana
partridge posture

salabhasana
locust posture

anantasana
side-lying stretch

supta vajrasana
supine thunderbolt posture

adho mukha svanasana
downward-facing dog posture

uttihita trikonasana
extended triangle posture

utkatasana
squatting posture

sarvangasana **shoulder stand**
(increases the body's metabolic rate while in the posture)

routine for children (15 minutes)

Children have an incredible amount of energy, and yoga will help to harness it productively. They are also naturally flexible and have a good sense of balance. Hence, children are generally able to adopt many of the asanas with relative ease. Use gentle physical guidance to correct them, never forcing the muscles and joints. At first, as a child may find it difficult to sit still, use dynamic practice. Channel the child's imagination, for example, use animal noises when adopting asanas involving animal positions. If yoga is practiced through the childhood years, the body's muscles will retain their childhood elasticity into adulthood.

warm-ups: Shoulder rolls, Windmill, Hip rotation, Spinning, Rocking the body

A seed rests quietly under the warm soil.

The pitter-patter rain falls on the ground and the seed pops its head up from the ground.

start

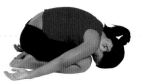

balasana
child's posture
page 56

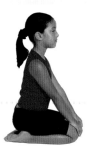

vajrasana
thunderbolt posture
page 51

The sun beams down on the sapling, making it grow upward.

The young tree spreads its roots to make it strong, ready to grow even bigger.

With more rain and sun the tree grows bigger and bigger, until it is a strong, tall tree.

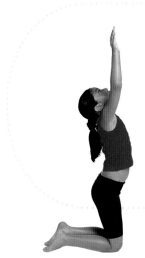

nagasana
raised serpent posture
page 83

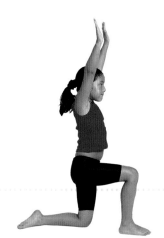

hanumanasana
hanuman posture
page 42

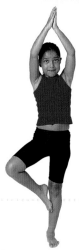

finish

vrksasana
tree posture
page 102

Purring softly, arch the back up and down like an elegant cat.

Lie still like a crocodile resting on a rock, basking in the warm sunshine.

Rise up like a proud and majestic cobra, holding still to observe the world.

start

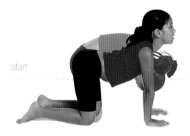

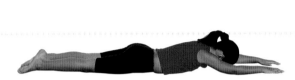

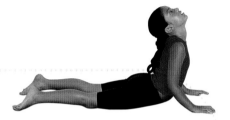

bilikasana
cat posture
pages 52–53

makarasana
crocodile posture
page 65

bhujangasana
cobra posture
page 73

Your legs are the wings of the butterfly, gently fluttering up and down.

Imagine a balloon in the chest, gently inflating as you breathe in and deflating as you breathe out.

Lie completely still and quietly listen to the gentle breath coming in and out.

finish

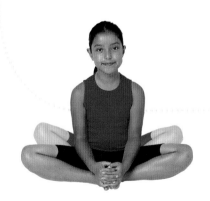

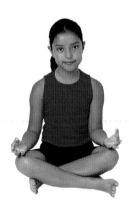

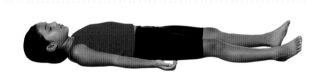

baddha konasana
cobbler posture
(follow with the butterfly posture)
page 60

pranayama in sukhasana
breathing in easy posture
page 27

savasana
corpse posture
page 91

routine for older people (20 minutes)

Yoga benefits all, regardless of age and ability. In the later years, the pace of life is slower and there may be more time to develop the body and mind. Dedicating a small period of the day to practicing yoga asanas will improve memory and concentration, increase energy levels, and develop a more positive and focused outlook on life. Meditation can help the person to become centered and generate an internal calmness. Awareness of the breath is increased and breathing becomes more efficient. The spine as it advances through the decades can be prone to contraction and will benefit from being stretched and extended. The muscles of the body as they are stretched will become toned. Postures that involve weight bearing through the bones of the limbs and joints will counter the reduction in bone density that is often prevalent in later life, particularly in postmenopausal women. At first, some asanas may be difficult to attain. Practice with a simpler variation (this has been shown for some of the asanas) and in time incorporate the more difficult asanas into the routine. If breathlessness occurs, then relax in Savasana until the breathing becomes steady. Practice after a warm bath so that the stiffness in the joints and muscles is reduced.

warm-ups: Neck stretch, Sitting arm and neck stretch, Knee-to-head in supine position, Rocking the body

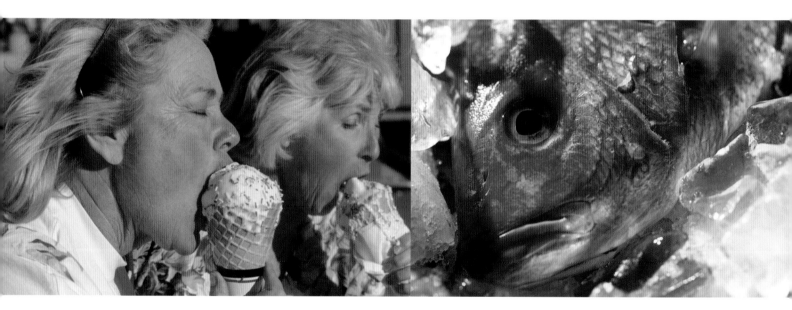

Staying healthy as an older adult doesn't have to be difficult. Here are some other ways that you can help yourself:

get out and about

Retirement is a good opportunity to pursue a more active social life. Meeting new people is an excellent way to stimulate the mind and keep alert. There are many activities that you can engage in, for example, walking in parks, visiting museums, and attending classes. It is never too late to take up new pursuits.

dietary considerations

Eating lots of fresh fruits and vegetables, which are rich in vitamins, will help to maintain healthy bones and tissues. Folic acid, magnesium, vitamin B6, and B12, found in green vegetables such as spinach, are considered boosters of our natural immunity. They are also thought to help protect against coronary disease. Vitamin E, found in nuts, seeds, whole grains, and egg yolks, is believed to help slow down or prevent mental decline.

positive thinking

A positive outlook on life helps you stay healthy. So much of your health as an older adult depends on your approach and mental attitude. If you look on the positive side, it's likely that your body will feel good about itself, too.

above left: A good social life can bring mental and physical benefits to older adults.
above right: Oily fish can help loosen up stiff joints.

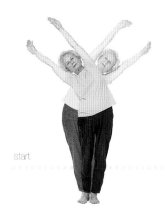

start

urdhva hastottasana
upstretched arms posture

page 40

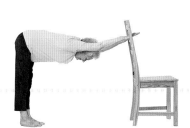

ardha uttanasana
half forward bend

page 77

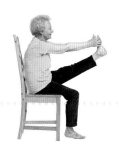

uttihita hasta padangusthasana
extended hand-to-big-toe posture
(in sitting)

page 105

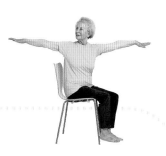

maricyasana
spinal twist in sitting

page 110

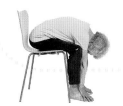

uttanasana
forward bend, sitting on a chair

page 78

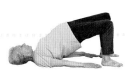

setu bandhasana
bridge posture

page 96

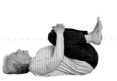

pavanmuktasana
wind-relieving posture

page 92

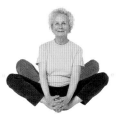

baddha konasana
cobbler posture
(follow with butterfly posture)

page 60

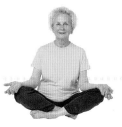

pranayama in sukhasana
breathing in easy posture

page 27

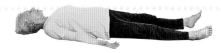

savasana
corpse posture

page 91

finish

routine for back relief (20 minutes)

Back pain is a common condition that can arise from poor posture, weakness in the back and abdominal muscles, excessive lifting, and trauma. In many occupations, back problems are considered a professional hazard. Health care professionals, builders, truck drivers, supermarket checkout persons, etc., will often use one side of the body more than the other and not be aware that they are compensating with movements in the opposite direction. Yoga asanas counteract contortional stress to the back muscles and spine and train the body to become more aware of posture and breathing patterns. Hence, yoga goes a long way to relieving the pain or alleviating it completely. However, if spinal curvature, a slipped disk, spinal arthritis, or inflammation is the root cause of back pain, then postures must be undertaken under the guidance of a yoga therapist.

warm-ups: Upper arm stretch, Sitting arm and neck stretch, Front-to-side leg raise, and Thigh stretch

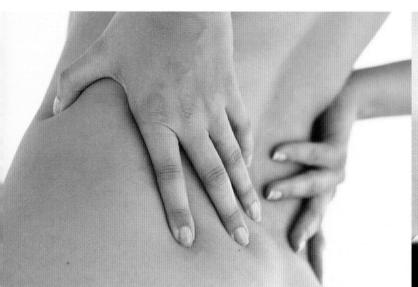
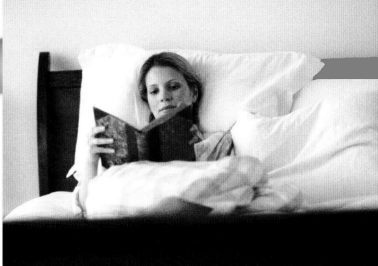

daily back care

This kind of yoga routine is crucial in caring for your back. But there are lots of other things you can do to help prevent back pain:

lifting

When lifting heavy objects, never bend from the waist. Bend your knees and squat next to the object, then lift. This way, you're allowing the strength of your leg muscles to bear the weight, rather than pulling down on the back. Hold the object close to your body and try not to twist your body around.

sitting pretty

None of us were made to sit at a desk for hours on end, but that's what most of us do these days. Make sure your chair and desk are ergonomic. This can be as simple as bringing a cushion to work to

put behind your back when you're sitting in front of the computer. Take time out to interlock the fingers and stretch the arms above the head.

back in bed

If you've recently developed back pain, it may be that you need to buy a new mattress for your bed. There are some good orthopaedic mattresses available, but the main thing is to make sure that your mattress is nice and firm, giving your back the support it needs.

above left: Back pain affects millions of people, young and old, and even small twinges can be a warning of worse pain to come—so listen to your body.
above right: Investing in a firm mattress for your bed is one of the best treats you can give your back.

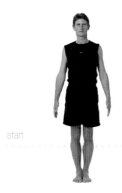

start

tadasana

mountain posture

page 39

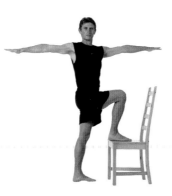

maricyasana

spinal twist in standing

page 109

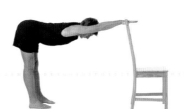

ardha uttanasana

half forward bend

page 77

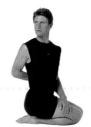

parivrtta vajrasana

thunderbolt twist

page 112

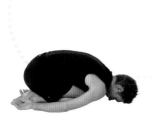

balasana

child's posture

page 56

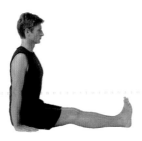

dandasana

staff posture

page 58

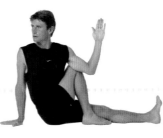

maricyasana

lateral sitting twist

page 110

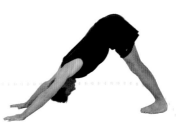

adho mukha svanasana

downward-facing dog posture

page 66

finish

makarasana

crocodile posture

page 65

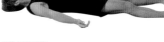

savasana

corpse posture

page 91

routine for detox (20 minutes)

The use of stimulants such as tobacco, alcohol, coffee, tea, etc. has a stressful effect on the mind and body, and places considerable strain on the internal organs that work to remove the toxins from the system. The consumption of processed food, refined white sugars, additives, etc., also places a strain on the internal abdominal organs. Poor diet and reliance on stimulants will slow down the body's processes and reduce energy levels. The practice of yoga asanas, pranayama, and meditation will build an inner strength to overcome the desire for and dependency on stimulants. This basic yoga routine performed regularly will enhance the body's natural cleansing process. As the mind and body are purified, there is increased awareness of the harmful effects of stimulants, and new patterns of healthier living will develop.

warm-ups: Neck stretch, Shoulder rolls, Upper arm stretch, Sitting arm and Neck stretch, Sun salutation (2 cycles)

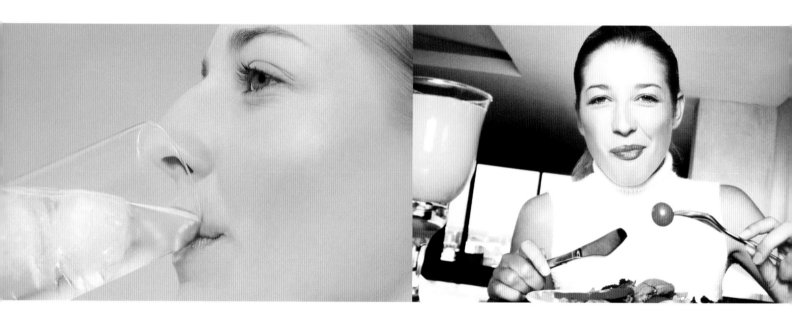

What else can you do to clear out your system? Some detox methods can be severe, but there are gentler ways of detoxing:

• Drink lots of water (plain water, rather than sparkling).
• Avoid caffeine and alcohol. If you have a blender, make yourself some pure fruit smoothies, as these can be a great source of vitamins, fiber, and energy-boosting potassium.
• Take invigorating showers. While you're in there, give yourself an all-over body scrub. This will slough off dead skin cells, boost your circulation, and leave you feeling extremely alert.
• A facial steam is easy to do at home and sweats out all the grime and dirt that clogs up your pores.

above left: Drink at least eight glasses of water as part of a detox program.
above right: Eating lots of salad will provide you with water, fiber, and vitamins.

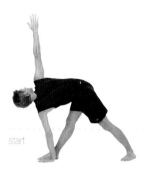

start

parivrtta trikonasana
reverse triangle posture

page 44

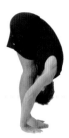

uttanasana
forward bend

page 78

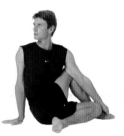

ardha matsyendrasana
half twist in sitting

page 111

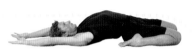

supta vajrasana
supine thunderbolt posture

page 84

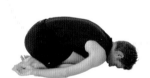

balasana
child's posture

page 56

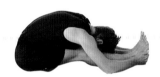

paschimo hanasana
forward bend in sitting

page 87

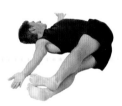

jathara parivartanasana
belly-turning posture

pages 114–115

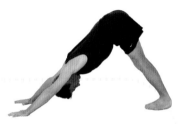

adho mukha svanasana
downward-facing dog posture

page 66

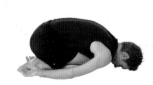

balasana
child's posture

page 56

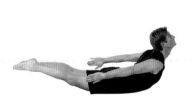

salabhasana
locust posture

pages 70–71

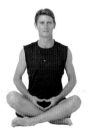

pranayama in sukhasana
breathing in easy posture

page 27

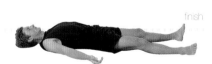

finish

savasana
corpse posture

page 91

preparing for meditation **in lotus position (15 minutes)**

Padmasana, or the Lotus posture, is the classical posture used for meditation purposes. The feet and legs are firmly locked in position to give a stabilizing base to the lower body. The spine is held erect and the body's energy is able to flow toward the brain. It is probably the most difficult posture to achieve. However, this program is designed to develop flexibility in the knees and ankles. With regular practice of the postures contained in this program, the seemingly impossible Lotus posture will be achieved.

warm-ups: Upper arm stretch, Hip rotation, Front-to-side leg raise, Thigh stretch, Leg pendulum, Rocking the body

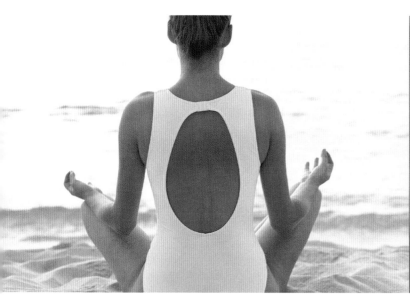
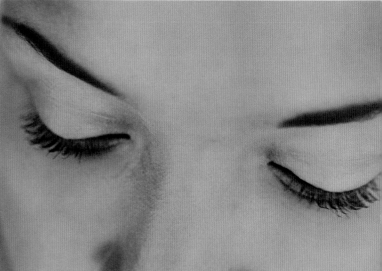

This routine will help the mind and body prepare for meditation. Sit in a quiet, warm, and dimly lit room. Close the eyes and use the breath to focus inward. Chanting is a good way of beginning meditation as it helps to develop an awareness of inner peace.

soham ("I am that which I am") chanting
The sound "Soham" is derived from the natural sound of breathing. "So" is the sound made when inhaling and "ham" is the sound made when exhaling. Repeat for 5–10 minutes, feeling the sound reverberating inside the body. Then hear the sound, without vocalizing, for 2–3 minutes. Feel the calming effect of this mantra.

above left: With enough practice, you can learn to meditate wherever you are.
above right: Closing your eyes allows you to concentrate on your inner self during meditation.

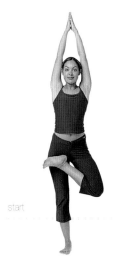

start

vrkasana
tree posture

page 102

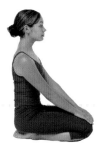

vajrasana
thunderbolt posture

page 51

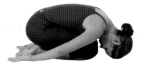

supta vajrasana
supine thunderbolt posture

page 84

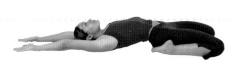

balasana
child's posture

page 56

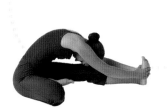

janu sirshasana
head-to-knee posture

page 88

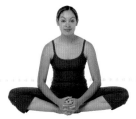

baddha konasana
cobbler posture

(follow with the butterfly posture)

page 60

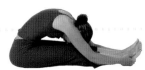

paschimottanasana
forward bend in sitting

page 87

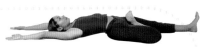

supta vrkasana
supine tree posture

page 99

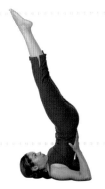

sarvangasana
shoulder stand

page 117

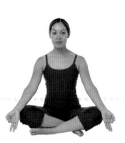

pranayama in sukhasana
breathing in easy posture

page 27

finish

routine for jet lag (20 minutes)

The number of people traveling long distances by air has increased steeply and is now a common part of our modern life. Air travel can have a very stressful effect on the body. Before the flight, there may be the anxiety of getting to the airport on time or a genuine fear of flying. During the flight, the body is cramped in one position for a long period, resulting in joint stiffness. On night flights, sleep can be interrupted and uncomfortable. After the flight, the body will have to adjust to a new environment that can have different temperature levels, oxygen levels due to a new altitude, culture, language, etc. Movement across time zones means that the internal body clock needs to be readjusted. Yoga asanas performed before, during, and after the flight will help to considerably reduce the stresses that air travel places on the body. Before the flight, practice the energizing dynamic routine to increase energy levels. During the flight, even when sitting, pay attention to posture and breathing. Use the aisle, when meals or drinks are not being served, to stretch the legs and arms. This is now recommended by many airlines for long flights. Simply standing in Tadasana will bring realignment to the body. After the flight, this simple routine can integrate the senses and replenish the body's energies.

warm-ups: Neck stretch, Shoulder rolls, Upper arm stretch, Hip rotation, Front-to-side leg raise, Thigh stretch, Leg pendulum, Sitting arm and neck stretch

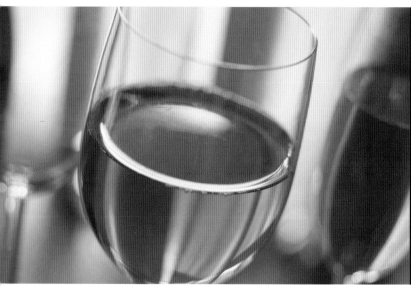
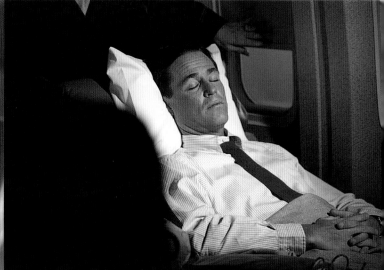

during the flight:

1 Wear layers of clothing so that they can be easily removed or put on depending on your body temperature.

2 Remove shoes and stretch toes and legs frequently.

3 Stand up often and stretch the limbs. Extend up on toes to stretch legs.

4 Drink plenty of water during the flight.

5 Spend a few minutes of each hour focusing on the breath and calming the mind.

above left: Avoid drinking alcohol on long flights, as it will add to the dehydration.

above right: Use a pillow to give the head a comfortable resting position.

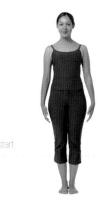

start

tadasana

mountain posture

page 39

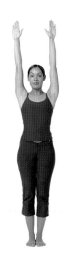

urdhva hastottasana

upstretched arms posture

page 40

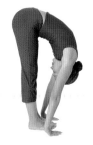

uttihita trikoasana

extended triangle posture

page 43

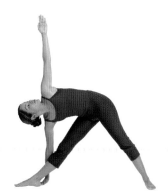

uttanasana

forward bend

page 78

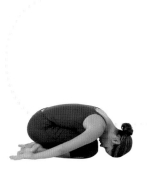

balasana

child's posture

page 56

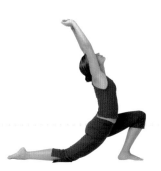

anjaneyasana

crescent moon posture

page 86

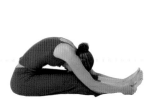

paschimottasana

forward bend in sitting

page 87

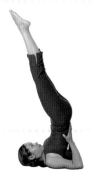

sarvangasana

shoulder stand

page 117

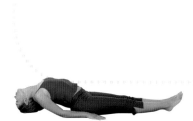

matsyasana

fish posture

page 97

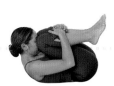

pavanmuktasana

wind-relieving posture

page 92

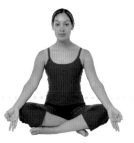

pranayama in sukhasana

breathing in easy posture

page 27

finish

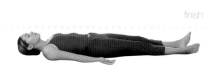

savasana

corpse posture

page 91

routine for runners (15 minutes)

In running, the knees are repetitively flexed to varying degrees. The bones and muscles are jarred in up-and-down movements. Leg muscles are disproportionally used in running, which can cause shortening of the tendons. Even with sensible footwear and soft surfaces, this action can place strain on the knee and ankle joints. Practicing yoga for a few minutes after a running session will rejuvenate the joints, massage the heart, and give a holistic stretch to all the leg muscles.

level: Intermediate

warm-ups: Neck stretch, Windmill, Front-to-side leg raise, Thigh stretch, Leg pendulum, Head-to-knee in supine, Rocking the body

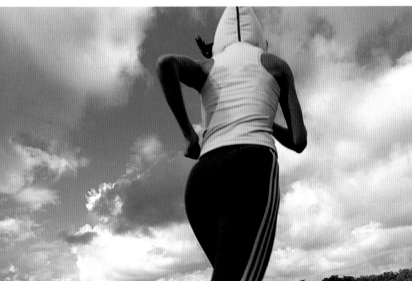 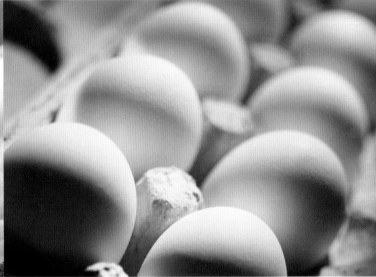

running safety

1 Running is a great way to keep fit, but as with all forms of exercise, you must also look after yourself.

2 Make sure you wear the right footwear. Tennis shoes don't give you the support you need—buy proper running shoes. And when you've bought them, give yourself lots of time to break them in. Don't run a marathon wearing a new pair of running shoes—your feet will be covered in blisters.

3 Give yourself lots of time to warm up and cool down before and after going for a run. Running is an extreme form of exercise and you'll suffer from a lot of pain and stiffness if you don't take the time to stretch your muscles.

4 If you're out running on country lanes or urban roads, make sure drivers and pedestrians can see you. Wear reflective clothing and keep an eye out for traffic and other people.

above left: Running is one of the most convenient forms of exercise.

above right: Calcium-rich foods are important for runners, as they help to maintain your bones and protect against osteoporosis.

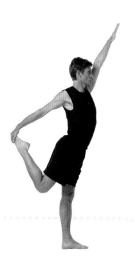

start

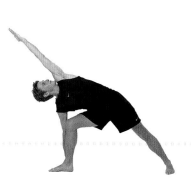

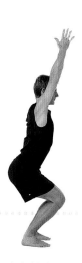

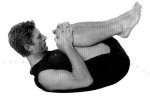

tadasana
mountain posture
page 39

uttihita trikonasana
extended triangle posture
page 43

sahaj uktatasana
chair posture
page 41

natarajasana
dancer posture
page 103

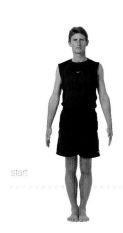

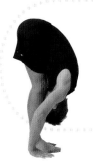

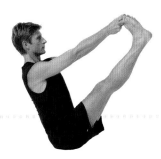

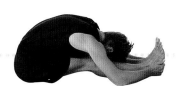

uttanasana
forward bend standing
page 78

ubhaya hasta padangusthasana
sitting balance posture
page 107

paschimottanasana
forward bend in sitting
page 87

pavanmuktasana
wind relieving posture
page 92

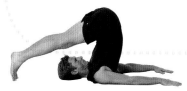

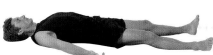

finish

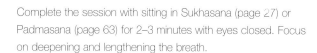

halasana
plow posture
page 118

savasana
corpse posture
page 91

Complete the session with sitting in Sukhasana (page 27) or
Padmasana (page 63) for 2–3 minutes with eyes closed. Focus
on deepening and lengthening the breath.

routine for cyclists (15 minutes)

In cycling, the repetitive movements involve flexion of the knees, but no counteractive extension. As the action does not allow the legs to be fully extended, the muscles employed in the movement are not fully stretched. Hence regular cyclists are prone to shortening of the hamstrings found at the back of the legs. Yoga postures carried out before and after a bicycle ride will help to counter the effects and maintain the tone and elasticity of the muscles. Even if it is not possible to carry out all the postures in a quiet room, some simple stretches can be done anywhere.

level: Intermediate

warm-ups: Neck stretch, Windmill, Front-to-side leg raise, Thigh stretch, Leg pendulum

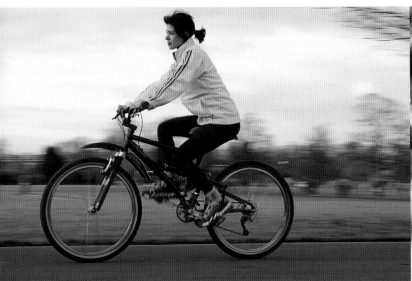
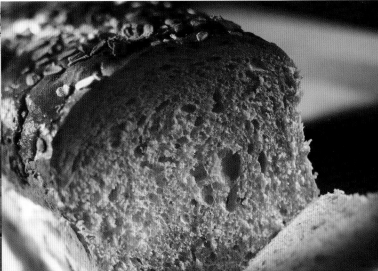

cycling safety

1 Bicycling is one of the most efficient and convenient forms of exercise. But you have to be careful, particularly if cycling in an urban environment.

2 Wear a cycling helmet—protecting the head is important in the event that you fall off your bicycle.

3 Make yourself seen. If cycling at night, always use your lights—without them, you're virtually invisible. Buy yourself a reflective vest and wear it!

4 Plan your route. With a bit of forward thinking, it's easy to plan a backstreet route so that you avoid the main, heavily-congested roads. Get out a map and look for parks, bike paths, and side streets. Your journey will be a lot more pleasant—and safer.

above left: Cycling is a good form of cardiovascular exercise.
above right: Bread is a good source of complex carbohydrates—essential for the slow release of energy.

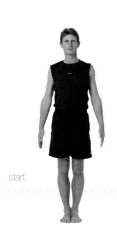

start

tadasana
mountain posture

page 39

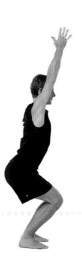

virabhadrasana
warrior posture

page 47

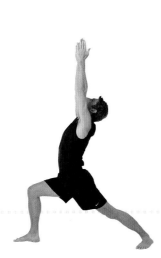

uktatasana
chair posture

page 41

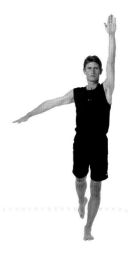

asvattasana
holy fig tree posture

page 101

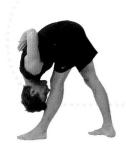

parsvottanasana
sideways forward stretch

page 80

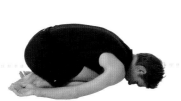

balasana
child's posture

page 56

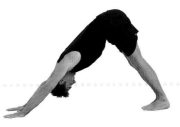

adho mukha svanasana
downward-facing dog posture

page 66

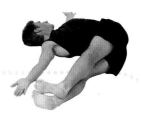

jathara parivartanasana
belly-turning posture

page 114

finish

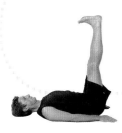

udhitta padasana
raised leg posture

page 93

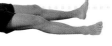
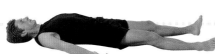

savasana
corpse posture

page 91

Complete the session with sitting in Sukhasana (page 27) or Padmasana (page 63) for 2–3 minutes with eyes closed. Focus on deepening and lengthening the breath.

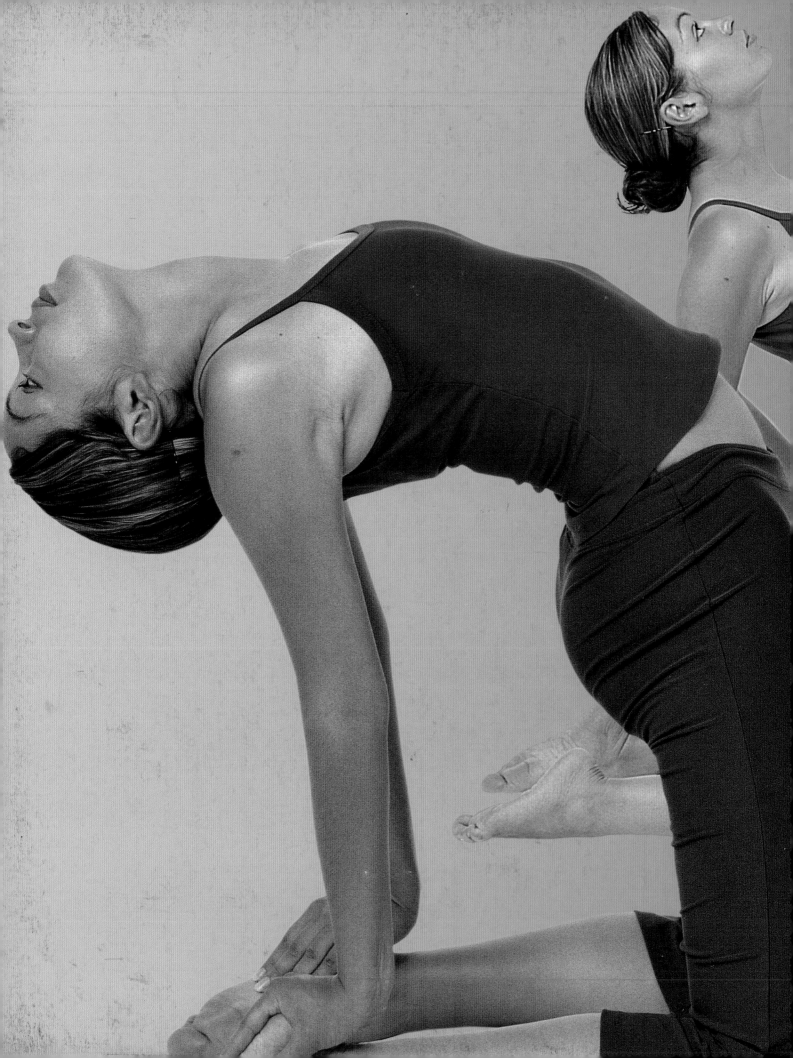

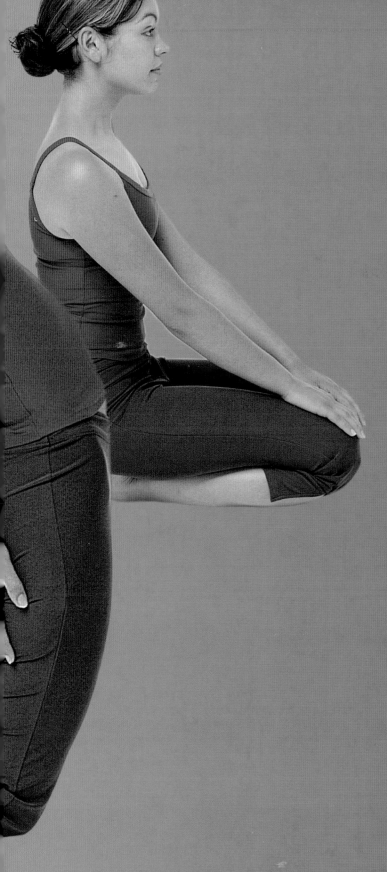

yoga for
common problems

yoga for common problems

Consult a yoga therapist for further guidance on postures suitable for your condition. Combine practice of above with alternative systems such as homeopathy. Follow a good diet, with a high intake of water, fruit, nuts, and fresh vegetables.

asthma

Over the last few decades, there has been a marked increase in the incidence of asthma. During an asthma attack the lungs' airways swell up and can produce mucus, making it difficult to catch your breath or—in the most severe cases—to breathe at all. For asthma sufferers it is beneficial to take up yoga. In particular, the controlled breathing exercises of Pranayama will help to strengthen the lungs, and the deep breathing exercises will help them compensate for the shallow breathing that accompanies asthma attacks.

recommended asanas	pranayama
uttanasana forward bend	kapalabhati cleansing breath
ardha chakrasana half wheel posture	anuloma viloma alternate nostril breathing
sarvangasana shoulder stand	
pavanmuktasana wind-relieving posture	
dhanaurasana bow posture	
savasana corpse posture	

high blood pressure

There are very few obvious symptoms of high blood pressure. This is why it is so important to make sure that your doctor regularly takes your blood pressure—particularly if you have a history of this illness in your family. High blood pressure equates to heart muscles working harder to pump blood around the body, increasing the risk of heart attacks. Reducing body weight and eating a healthy diet, low in salt and carbohydrates and high in minerals and vitamins, will help to reduce high blood pressure. The gentle approach of yoga means you can avoid the danger of overstimulating the heart. Yoga is energy-conserving; the postures use minimum energy for maximum stretch. Always check with your doctor before beginning any type of exercise.

recommended asanas	pranayama
halasana plow posture	kapalabhati cleansing breath
sarvangasana shoulder stand	
paschimottanasana forward bend in sitting	
savasana corpse posture	

circulatory problems

There are several causes of bad circulation—it may be hereditary, a symptom of bad diet or lifestyle, or a side effect of other illnesses such as diabetes or heart disease. Some of the signs of bad circulation include cold hands and feet, numbness, dizziness, and decreased urine output. The stretching and muscular stimulation derived from yoga can help to dilate the blood vessels and increase the blood circulation to the extremities. As circulation is improved from the practice of yoga, the skin is nourished, the brain becomes alert, and energy levels are increased.

recommended asanas	pranayama
hanumanasana hanuman posture	anuloma viloma alternate nostril breathing
garudasana eagle posture	
bakasana crane posture	

constipation

Constipation occurs when the bowels absorb water out of the feces and back into the body, making the feces hard and dry, and difficult to pass. Yoga goes a long way to assisting the problem of constipation as it massages the abdominal organs. The stretching and compression gained in postures helps to improve function of organs involved in the digestive process. Toxins are eliminated as the blood flow to the organs is improved. Postures in prone position are particularly effective for relieving constipation.

recommended asanas	pranayama
parivrtta parsvakonasana **reverse lateral angle stretch**	anuloma viloma **alternate nostril breathing**
prasarita padottanasana **standing-wide forward bend**	
utkatasana **squatting posture**	
balasana **child's posture**	
pavanmuktasana **wind-relieving posture**	
adho mukha svanasana **downward-facing dog posture**	
bhujangasana **cobra posture**	
halasana **plow posture**	

fatigue

In our modern hectic lifestyle, it is easy to forget the needs of the body. Missing breakfast, overusing stimulants such as coffee and tea, not getting enough sleep, recovering from illness, emotional pressure, stress at work, and poor breathing patterns all result in low energy levels. But one of the best ways of countering fatigue is by looking after your body. Even the preliminary warm-up exercises of yoga help to stretch your body and boost energy levels, while simple posture exercises can help "remind" your body about itself and counter feelings of sluggishness. If you practice the nighttime yoga routine, you'll get a good night's sleep and fatigue should be banished!

recommended asanas	pranayama
sarvangasana **shoulder stand**	kapalabhati **cleansing breath**
halasana **plow posture**	ujjayi **victorious breath**
paschimottanasana **forward bend in sitting**	anuloma viloma **alternate nostril breathing**
uttanasana **forward bend**	
sirshasana **headstand**	
savasana **corpse posture**	

fertility problems

Infertility affects one in seven couples. Treatment is often difficult and highly stressful emotionally. Stress can have a significant impact on fertility and it is now widely recommended that people take up an activity such as yoga because of its well-known benefits as a relaxing form of exercise. As well as reducing stress, yoga has a beneficial effect on improving the function of the reproductive organs. Your yoga session may become the one time of the day when you are able to stop thinking about having a baby and start concentrating on yourself.

recommended asanas	pranayama
baddha konasana **cobbler posture**	sithali **cooling breath**
ustrasana **camel posture**	
adho mukha svanasana **downward-facing dog posture**	
matsyasana **fish posture**	

hay fever

As summer arrives and the pollen count increases, huge numbers of people are thrown into misery as their allergies produce itchy, watery eyes and nose, sneezing, coughing, and in severe cases, difficulty breathing. The problem can be exacerbated if you're living in an urban area, where pollens and molds are trapped by the environment. The breathing exercises are particularly beneficial for "reopening" the lungs and cleansing the nasal and throat airways.

recommended asanas	pranayama
sasamgasana hare posture	kapalabhati cleansing breath

hemorrhoids

Hemorrhoids affect a large part of the population. They are swollen tissues that bulge into the anus, and can be itchy and painful, sometimes bleeding. Specific yoga postures can help to stretch and energize the pelvic floor muscles and give relief to the painful effects of hemorrhoids.

recommended asanas	pranayama
sarvangasana shoulder stand	kapalabhati cleansing breath

headaches

From the occasional headache to severe and debilitating migraines, we all suffer from headaches at one time or another. Headaches can be caused by a myriad of reasons: emotional stress, dehydration, food allergies, tension, or even just the way you're sitting. What's most important is what you do once a headache starts, and one of the best things is to place yourself in a relaxing and stress-free environment, away from bright lights and noise. Yoga postures can be very beneficial to relieving a headache. Select postures that are comfortable and enable the body and mind to be relaxed.

recommended asanas	pranayama
balasana child's posture	kapalabhati cleansing breath
savasana corpse posture	ujjayi victorious breath
makarasana crocodile posture	

insomnia

Insomnia can be a frustrating condition to suffer—even if you're desperately tired you still can't fall asleep and/or stay asleep. A lack of routine, anxiety, or depression can all be causes—as can exercising or eating too late at night. Yoga postures and breathing exercises can help to relieve the tension held in the body and allow the mind to become calmer. The mind and body will then welcome the transition from wakefulness to sleep. If you are suffering from insomnia, you'll find that yoga can really help. A good evening session of yoga will help you relax and unwind. It's often the case that people can't sleep because they haven't managed to switch their mind off by the time they go to bed. Any simple yoga routine, which forces you to focus only on the present, will enable you to clear your head of clutter—and get a good night's sleep. Even if you wake in the middle of the night you can still practice some of the breathing routines without even getting out of bed.

recommended asanas	pranayama
sirshasana headstand	kapalabhati cleansing breath
sarvangasana shoulder stand	anuloma viloma alternate nostril breathing
paschimottanasana forward bend in sitting	

kidney problems

The kidneys are located near the middle of your back. They are bean-shaped organs about the size of your fist. They filter blood and water for waste, which is taken away in urine. The biggest causes of kidney problems are high blood pressure and diabetes. A blow to the kidneys or taking too many painkillers can also damage the kidneys. In the early stages of kidney disease, you may not even realize that anything is wrong. This is why it is so important to ensure your lifestyle and diet are both healthy, so that problems don't develop in the first place. Yoga postures help to improve the function of the kidneys, increasing blood flow and eliminating toxins.

recommended asanas	pranayama
savasana **corpse posture** supta vajrasana **supine thunderbolt posture** salabhasana **locust posture**	sithali **cooling breath**

memory problems

When so many demands are being made on us by the modern, busy lifestyle it's all too easy for the brain to lose its focus and for you to start forgetting things. A yoga session may be your only chance in the day to take time out and take stock. Yoga encourages you to clear your head and focus only on the movements and exercises you're doing. This in turn allows you to unconsciously rearrange your mindset and refocus the brain and give clarity of thought—so that you return to the world clear-headed and alert.

recommended asanas	pranayama
vrksasana **tree posture** karnapidasana **ear-closing posture** sirshasana **headstand** savasana **corpse posture**	kapalabhati **cleansing breath**

varicose veins

Varicose veins in your legs have a blue appearance with bulges and knots in the vein that distort the surface of the skin. They can ache or be painful and many people are concerned by their unsightly appearance. The reason people get varicose veins is because of faulty valves in the vein system, which means the veins are less efficient at carrying blood around the body. Hence blood pools or flows the wrong way, causing the veins to swell. If you suffer from varicose veins, then yoga can help relieve some of the symptoms. Exercises that encourage you to raise your legs above your head help take the pressure off these weak veins and yoga exercises in general help to invigorate your circulation. Inverted postures are particularly useful for aiding drainage.

recommended asanas	pranayama
sarvangasana **shoulder stand** matsyasana **fish posture**	sithali **cooling breath**

glossary

Adho-mukha facing downward

Advita nondualistic

Ahimsa the doctrine of nonviolence

Ajna Chakra energy center between the eyebrows

Akasha ether or primordial substance that pervades the entire universe

Anahata Chakra energy center at the heart

Anamika ring finger

Ananda bliss or divine happiness

Ananta cosmic serpent or eternity

Anga body

Angi fire element

Angula finger or thumb

Angustha big toe or thumb

Anja form

Anuloma with order

Ardha half

Asana steady pose or posture; the third path of Patanjali's eight-limbed yoga

Ashtanga eight limbs of Patanjali's yoga

Atharva Veda knowledge of mystical incantations

Atman human soul or spirit

Aum omnipresence

Ayama stretch

Ayurveda traditional Indian healing system

Avirati sensuality

Baddha restrain

Bala infant or child

Bandha lock or bond—relates to contracting muscles to control the flow of prana

Baka crane

Bhagavad Gita divine song—relates to the dialog between Arjuna and Krishna

Bhakti devotion or adoration; Bhakti yoga is the practice of constant devotion to the divine

Bhati practice that brings lightness

Bhagavad divine one

Bhagavan god

Bharadvaja Indian sage

Bhaya Kumbhaka external breath retention

Bija seed

Bija-mantra the repetition of a Sanskrit syllable with pranayama to seed the growth of oneness

Brahmacharya self-control such as celibacy

Brahman the supreme being who represents the highest principle in the universe; the essence that permeates all existence

Brahmari bee

Buddhi intellect

Chakras wheel, referring to the revolving energy centers

Chandra the moon

Chitta consciousness

Danda a staff

Deva god

Dhanu bow

Dharana concentration—the sixth path of Patanjali's eight-limbed yoga

Dharma path taken in life, which can lead to a higher state of consciousness

Dhyana meditation—the seventh stage of Patanjali's eight-limbed yoga

Dola swing

Drashta seer or witness

Duhka pain or sorrow

Eka one or single

Ekagra concentrated or one-pointedness

Garuda eagle deity

Gita song

Go cow

Guna cosmic energy or quality of nature

Guru spiritual teacher

Hala plow

Hanuman the monkey warrior who served Rama in his battle against Ravana

Hasta the hand

Hatha "Ha" is the sun and "tha" is the moon. Hatha yoga is the balancing of the lunar and solar energies.

Himalayas mountain range in northern India

Ida energy channel also called 'chandra nadi' located on the left side of the body

Indra god of thunder, lightning, and rain

Isvara the supreme being; god

Jal water element

Jalandhara Bandha chin pressing against the breastbone to lock the airways

Janu knee

Japa repetitive mantra

Jathara abdomen

Jaya victory or conquest

Jivatma the individual soul

Jnana Yoga the path of wisdom or knowledge of the self

Kailasa the mountain abode of Lord Shiva

Kaivalya final emancipation; fourth and final path in the Yoga Sutras

Kali Yuga the age of destruction

Kanishthika little finger

Kapala skull

Karma the cosmic law of action; every action has consequences; Karma Yoga is the practice of right actions without gain

Karna the ear

Klesas pain or suffering

Kona angle

Kriyas duties

Kshatriyas warrior caste

Kundalini the dormant serpent energy at the base of the spine, which, when awakened, rises up through the chakras, uniting with the universal soul

Lingam phallus

Madhyama middle finger

Manas mind

Mandala circle; symbol of unity used for meditation

Manipura Chakra energy center at the navel

Mantras sacred Sanskrit syllables repeated during meditation

Marichi name of a sage

Matsya fish

Matsyendra one of the first teachers of yoga

Maya illusion

Moksha attainment of liberation or release from the cycle of births

Mudra seal by muscular contraction

Mukta liberated

Mukha face

Muladhara chakra root center at the base of the spine

Nadi energy channel in the subtle body

Nama name

Namaskar greeting

Nandi shiva's bull

Nataraj Lord of the dance or shiva

Nava boat

Neya time passed

Ni down

Nirvana transcendental state of bliss

Nirvikalpa free from distinctions

Niyama self-purification; second stage of Patanjali's eight-limbed yoga

Ojas physic power developed through certain yogic practises

Om the sacred syllable or universal sound

Pada foot or leg

Padangustha big toe

Padma lotus

Parigha bar for securing gate

Paripurna complete or entire

Parvati female consort of Lord Shiva

Parivrtta rotated or reversed

Paschima back

Patanjali founder of the eight limbs of yoga

Pavan wind

Pida pressure

Pingala energy channel located on the right side of the body

Prana the cosmic life force

Pranayama yogic breathing exercises for control and regulation of breath—the fourth stage of Patanjali's eight-limbed yoga

Pratyahara withdrawal of the mind from sensory and sensual experiences; the fifth stage of Patanjali's eight-limbed yoga

Puraka inhalation

Rahasya secrets

Raja king

Raja yoga mastery of the mind to attain liberation

Rajasic one of the three gunas; rich or royal

Rechaka exhalation

Rig Veda knowledge of hymns

Sadanga Yoga the six limbs of yoga contained in *Hatha Yoga Pradipika*

Sahasrara Chakra energy center at the cerebrum

Salabha locust

Sadhanas disciplines of attaining a spiritual goal

Samadhi the final self-realization or union of the individual consciousness with cosmic consciousness

Sama Veda knowledge of melodious chants

Samskara mental impressions

Sattvic one of the three gunas: purity, intelligence, illumination

Sava corpse

Setu bridge

Setu-bandha the construction of a bridge

Siddhis powers of the soul; attained through yogic disciplines

Sitali cool

Shakti female creative power and strength

Soham "I am that"; the unconscious breath sound uttered by all living creatures

Sudras caste of servants and laborers

Supta sleeping

Surya the sun

Sushumna the main energy channel located along the length of the spine

Sutra condensed literature

Svana dog

Swadhisthana Chakra sacral energy center

Tada mountain

Tantra practice of attaining liberation by unifying male and female energies

Tapas austere practices

Tat twam asi "thou that art"

Tamasic one of the three gunas; rancid or decaying

Trikona triangle

Ubhaya both

Uddiyana retraction of the abdomen

Ujjayi pranayama technique

Upanisad philosophical doctrines of the Vedas; relating the true nature of the man

Urdhva raised or elevated

Ustra camel

Utthita extended

Vaisyas caste of merchants and farmers

Vajra a thunderbolt; weapon used by Lord Indra

Valmiki sage who wrote the epic Ramayana

Vedanta one of the six schools of Indian philosophy; at the end of the vedas

Viloma against order

Vishnu god of preservation

Vishuddha Chakra energy center at the throat

Yajur Veda knowledge of sacrifice

Yamas universal moral decrees of nonviolence, truthfulness, honesty, etc.—the first stage of Patanjali's eight-limbed yoga

Yoga union; refers to the various practices for attaining union between the self and the infinite

Yogi or Yogini one who practices yoga

recommended yoga organizations

USA

American Yoga Association
P.O. Box 19986
Sarasota
FL 34276
USA
Tel: (+1) 941 927 4977
Fax: (+1) 941 921 9844
E-mail: info@americanyogaassocaition.org
Website: www.americanyogaassociation.org

3HO Foundation *(Focuses on Kundalini Yoga)*
Route 2
Box 4
Shady Lane
Espanola NM 87532
USA
Tel: (+1) 505 753 4988
Fax: (+1) 505 753 1999
E-mail: yogainfo@3ho.org
Website: www.3ho.org

Himalayan Institute
R.R. 1
P.O. Box 1127
Honesdale
PA 18431-9706
USA
Tel. (+1) 800 822 4547
Fax: (+1) 570 253 9078

Integral Yoga International
Satchidananda Ashram/Yogaville
R.R. 1 Box 1720
Buckingham
VA 23921
USA
Tel: (+1) 804 969 3121
Fax: (+1) 804 969 1303

White Lotus Yoga Foundation
2500 San Marcos Pass
Santa Barbara
CA 93105
USA
Tel: (+1) 805 964 1944
Fax: (+1) 805 964 9617
Website: www.whitelotus.org

International Association of Yoga Therapists
2400A County Center Drive
Santa Rosa
CA 95403
USA
Tel: (+1) 707 928 9898
Fax: (+1) 707 928 4738
E-mail: mail@iayt.org
Website: www.iayt.org

Yoga Alliance
120 South 3rd Avenue
West Reading
PA 19611
USA
Tel: (+1) 610 376 4421
E-mail: info@yogaalliance.org
Website: www.yogaalliance.org

International Association of Black Yoga Teachers
P.O. Box 360922
Los Angeles
CA 90036
USA
Tel: (+1) 213 833 6371

Yoga College of India World Headquarters
1862 S. LaCienega Blvd
Los Angeles
CA 90035
USA
Tel: (+1) 310 854 5800
Fax: (+1) 310 854 6200

Kripalu Centre for Yoga and Health
P.O. Box 793
Lenox
MA 01240
USA
Tel: (+1) 800 741 7353

Yoga Research and Education Center (YREC)
2400A County Center Drive
Santa Rosa
CA 95403
USA
Tel: (+1) 707 566 9000
E-mail: mail@yrec.org

Self-Realization Fellowship
3880 San Rafael Avenue
Dept 9W
Los Angeles
CA 90065-3298
USA
Tel: (+1) 323 225 2471
Fax: (+1) 323 225 5088
www.yogananda-srf.org

India

Purna Swasthya Yoga Therapy Clinic
1st Floor
Kalabhavan
Matthews Road
Mumbai 400004
India
E-mail: drpragnapatel@hotmail.com

Somatheeram Ayurvedic Beach Resort
Chowara P.O.
South of Kovalam
Trivandrum 695501
Kerala
South India
Tel: (+91) 471 268101
Fax: (+91) 471 267600
E-mail: somatheeram@vsnl.com
Website: www.somatheeram.com

Yoga-Ganga Centre for Yogic Studies
101 Old Rajpur
Dehradun
Uttranchal 248003
India
Tel: (+91) 135 733653 / 632793
Fax: (+91) 135632793
E-mail: yoganga@vsnl.com

Rama Yoga & Meditation Center
Thomson Villa
Near English Rose
Candolim Beach Road
Bardez
Goa
India 403515
E-mail: ramayogacenter@yahoo.com

UK

Yoga Therapy Centre
Royal London Homeopathic Hospital
4th Floor
60 Great Ormond Street
London
WC1N 3HR
UK
Tel: (+44) (0)20 7419 7195

Prison Phoenix Trust
P.O. Box 328
Oxford
OX2 7HF
UK
Tel: (+44) (0)1865 512521

The British Wheel Of Yoga
2 Jermyn Street
Sleaford
Lincs.
NG34 7RU
UK
Tel: (+44) (0)1529 306851
Fax: (+44) (0) 1529 303233
Website: www.bwy.org.uk

Sivananda Yoga Vedanta Centre
51 Felsham Road
London
SW15 1AZ
UK
Tel: (+44) (0)20 8780 0160

Bikram's Yoga College of India
173 Queen's Crescent
London
NW5 3DS
UK
Tel: (+44) (0)20 7692 6900

Viniyoga Britain
105 Gales Drive
Three Bridges
Crawley
West Sussex
RH10 1QD
UK

websites

www.ananda.org
details on the Ananda Community in California, plus home study course

www.santosha.com
philosophy on yoga, classes and events at the Yoga Anand Ashram in New York

www.sangamyoga.com
origins of Ashtanga yoga plus classes in UK

www.ashtanga.com
basic information on Vinyasa Ashtanga Yoga

www.sivananda.org
the American site for Sivananda yoga

www.ashtanga.org
resource site for Ashtanga Yoga

www.americanyogaassociation.org
free yoga lessons, online store selling books, videos, and cassettes for meditation

www.specialyoga.com
descibes the yoga education program developed by Sonia Sumar for children with special needs (e.g., Downs syndrome, cerebral palsy, autism)

www.bksiyengar.com
an introduction to Iyengar Yoga, including Association projects

www.expandinglight.org
information on Ananda Yoga; retreats and programs

www.himalayaninstitute.org
information on workshops and retreats; teachers training program; holistic health services; books, videotapes, and audiotapes

www.yoga.com
articles about Iyengar yoga

www.yogabasics.com
U.S. directory of teachers, information on asanas and pranayama

www.yogacards.com
directory of Hatha yoga postures with pictures

www.iyengar-yoga.com
comprehensive resource site on Iyengar Yoga—associations, centers, books, videos, etc.

www.yogadirectory.com
informative site, giving connections to many other yoga sites

www.kfoundation.org
information on the Krishnamurti Foundation, based in Hampshire, UK

www.yogaforbeginners.com
general introduction to different yoga styles, postures, and benefits

www.kripalu.com
information on activities, courses and retreats held at the Kripalu Center, USA

www.kundaliniyoga.com
information on Kundalini Yoga plus techniques on yoga cycles, teachers' directory, and teacher training

www.yogaworkshop.com
workshop information from Richard Freeman, the American teacher of Ashtanga Yoga

www.power-yoga.com
details on the Hard and Soft Ashtanga Yoga Institute based in New York and East Hampshire. Gives information on courses and vacations

www.yogaworld.org
Ramakrishna's site on techniques of meditation

www.ramakrishna.org
biography on Ramakrishna, program of the Ramakrishna-Vivekananda center of New York

www.youandmeyoga.com
training and teaching materials for staff, careers, and parents working with people with learning difficulties/disabilities

www.yrec.org
information on the Yoga research and Education Center with headquarters in Santa Rosa, California

yoga publications

books

The American Yoga Association's Easy Does It Yoga
Alice Christensen
A user-friendly book on yoga

Autobiography of a Yogi
Paramahansa Yogananda
An excellent book for any spiritual aspirant, this book clearly demonstrates the various forms of yoga and its simple beauty in attaining the divine.

Bhagavad Gita: A New Translation
Stephen Mitchell
An excellent book that is a good aid to learn Sanskrit, too. Based on the teachings of Shri Ramakrishna.

The Sivananda Companion to Yoga
Lucy Lidell
Book on Sivananda yoga

Dr. Dean Ornish's Program for Reversing Heart Disease
Dean Ornish, M.D.
Fascinating book on the therapeutic power of yoga

Hatha Yoga Pradipika
Pancham Sinh
Insightful reading

The Heart of Yoga
T. K. V. Desikachar
An in-depth book to gain a deeper understanding of yoga

Journey into Power
Baron Baptiste
Book on sculpting the ideal body and transforming attitudes

Light on Yoga
B. K. S. Iyengar
Great introductory book to Hatha yoga, with detailed postural techniques

Science of Breath
Swami Rama
This book encapsulates the powerful techniques for breathing

Yoga: A Gem for Women
Geeta S. Iyengar
Detailed descriptions with photographs to achieve perfection in the pose.

Yoga for the Special Child
Sonia Sumar, tr. Jeffrey Volk, Adriana Marusso
Special Yoga Publications, 1997
Yoga for the child with Downs syndrome, cerebral palsy, autism, attention deficit disorder, attention deficit hyperactivity disorder and learning disabilities

Yoga: The Path To Holistic Health
B. K. S. Iyengar
Another excellent book by the world renowned yoga teacher

The Yoga Sutras of Patanjali
Sri Swami Satchiananda
Integral Yoga Publications, 1990

journals and magazines

Yoga Community Newsletter
Yoga Voices
7173 Winter Rose Path
Columbia
MD 21045
USA
Tel: (+1) 410 290 5258
Fax: (+1) 410 290 7058
Email: evarose@yogavoices.com

Yoga International Magazine
(Published by the Himalayan Institute)
Rural Route 1
Box 1130
Honesdale
PA 18431-9718
USA
Tel: (+1) 570 253 6243
Fax: (+1) 570 253 6360

Yoga Journal
(Published by the California Yoga Teachers Association)
Editorial Department contact:
2054 University Avenue
Berkeley
CA 94704-1082
USA
Tel: (+1) 510 841 9200
Fax: (+1) 510 644 3101

Subscription Information, contact:
Yoga Journal
P.O. Box 469018
Escondido
CA 92046-9018
USA
Tel: (+1) 800 334 8152

Yoga World
The Yoga Research Center
P.O. Box 1386
Lower Lake
CA 95457
USA
Tel: (+1) 707 928 9898
Fax: (+1) 707 928 4738

Yoga & Health
21 Caburn Crescent
Lewes
East Sussex
BN7 1NR
UK

index